Photobiomodulation Therapy in Oral Medicine

Alan Roger Santos-Silva
Ana Gabriela Costa Normando
César Augusto Migliorati
Mariana de Pauli Paglioni
Editors

Aljomar José Vechiato Filho
Thaís Cristina Esteves-Pereira
Associate Editors

Photobiomodulation Therapy in Oral Medicine

Evidence-based Clinical Protocols

Springer

Editors
Alan Roger Santos-Silva
Oral Diagnosis Department
Piracicaba Dental School, University of Campinas
Piracicaba, SP, Brazil

Ana Gabriela Costa Normando
Oral Diagnosis Department
Piracicaba Dental School, University of Campinas
Piracicaba, SP, Brazil

César Augusto Migliorati
Department of Oral and Maxillofacial Diagnostic Sciences, College of Dentistry
University of Florida
Gainesville, FL, USA

Mariana de Pauli Paglioni
Oral Diagnosis Department
Piracicaba Dental School, University of Campinas
Piracicaba, SP, Brazil

Associate Editors
Aljomar José Vechiato Filho
Dental Oncology Service
São Paulo State Cancer Institute
University of São Paulo Medical School
São Paulo, SP, Brazil

Thaís Cristina Esteves-Pereira
Oral Diagnosis Department, Piracicaba Dental School, University of Campinas
Piracicaba, SP, Brazil

ISBN 978-3-031-85047-9 ISBN 978-3-031-85048-6 (eBook)
https://doi.org/10.1007/978-3-031-85048-6

This Springer imprint is published by the registered company Springer Nature Switzerland AG
The registered company address is: Gewerbestrasse 11, 6330 Cham, Switzerland

Oral Medicinists should strive to provide state-of-the-science care that safely enhances clinical outcomes in patients while reducing toxicity and the cost of treatment.

Adapted from Scully et al. Oral medicine (stomatology) across the globe: birth, growth, and future. Oral Surg Oral Med Oral Pathol Oral Radiol. 2016;121(2):149–157.e5.

Presentation

The primary aim of this book is to offer clinicians worldwide clear and concise guidelines for treating oral disorders using photobiomodulation therapy. It comprises over 20 chapters, each addressing a specific condition in a brief manner. To ensure accuracy, a structured literature search was conducted for each condition using MeSH terms and acronyms in MEDLINE via PubMed. The book prioritizes studies with higher levels of scientific evidence to support the protocols, including systematic reviews with meta-analyses, randomized clinical trials, and prospective cohorts. When high-quality studies were unavailable, case-control studies, case series, and case reports were used. Additionally, the expertise of our team has been integrated into the development of the book and the selection of qualified studies. For less explored themes, significant gaps may exist, making it challenging to provide objective guidelines.

At the end of each chapter, a table summarizes the photobiomodulation parameters. When a setup for both red and near-infrared (NIR) wavelengths is recommended, they are combined in a single entry. However, if the literature indicates that the disorder discussed in a specific chapter can be treated more effectively with red and NIR lights separately, the table includes distinct columns for each wavelength. The authors reviewed all chapters and included information only when there was consensus.

Foreword

It is a great pleasure and an honor to write the Foreword for this significant book on Photobiomodulation, conceived by my esteemed colleagues and friends in Oral Medicine, Alan Roger Santos-Silva and Cesar Migliorati.

For many years, I have known both within the "World of Light," witnessing the gradual and then explosive development of low-energy lasers and LEDs. This discipline, now termed "photobiomodulation," continues to uncover new clinical applications in medicine, dentistry, and well-being, with ever-increasing efficiency and scientific rigor.

As President of the World Association for Photobiomodulation Therapy (WALT) from 2021 to 2024, and with over 30 years of experience in developing this technique to manage the side effects of anticancer treatments, I have observed the remarkable evolution of photobiomodulation. Its technical advancements and effectiveness have been driven by a better understanding of its mechanisms and, more recently, by the precision and quality of dose delivery to target tissues. Photobiomodulation is now recognized as a well-developed technique with demonstrated efficacy and utility in addressing a wide variety of pathological processes, including pain, inflammation, and impaired wound healing. It has become particularly important in the field of Oral Medicine, where it is used to treat and manage various conditions affecting the oral cavity. Its noninvasive and nonthermal nature, combined with its therapeutic effects, has made it an invaluable tool for treating oral toxicities from cancer treatments and common oral mucosal diseases. By enhancing patient outcomes and improving quality of life, photobiomodulation represents a significant advancement in oral healthcare.

In this book, Dr. Santos-Silva and Dr. Migliorati infuse the field of Oral Medicine with infectious dynamism and boundless energy, presenting innovative protocols and insights for utilizing light and photobiomodulation. The advent of high-quality LEDs has significantly expanded the practical applications of this technology, and the authors leverage these advancements to explore its nearly limitless potential.

This meticulously written and highly informative book will resonate with a wide range of readers, far beyond the usual circle of light therapy enthusiasts. I wish the authors well-deserved success with this book and anticipate new, innovative protocols that will benefit all.

Nice, France René-Jean Bensadoun

Contents

Part I Photobiomodulation

1 **Basic Principles of Physics in Photobiomodulation** 3
Manoela Domingues Martins, Márcia Martins Marques, Thaís Cristina Esteves-Pereira, and Praveen R. Arany

2 **Understanding Dosimetry in Photobiomodulation Therapy** 11
Thaís Cristina Esteves-Pereira, Luiz Alcino Monteiro Gueiros, Praveen R. Arany, and Manoela Domingues Martins

3 **Equipment Quality Control and Selection** 17
Thaís Cristina Esteves-Pereira, Wilfredo Alejandro González-Arriagada, and João Adolfo Costa Hanemann

4 **Cross-Infection Control in Photobiomodulation Therapy** 25
Thaís Cristina Esteves-Pereira, João Adolfo Costa Hanemann, and René-Jean Bensadoun

5 **Safety and Adverse Effects in Photobiomodulation Therapy** 27
Thaís Cristina Esteves-Pereira, Thaís Bianca Brandão, René-Jean Bensadoun, Elisa Kauark Fontes, Mariana de Pauli Paglioni, and Alan Roger Santos-Silva

Part II Supportive Care in Cancer

6 **Oral Mucositis** 33
Ana Carolina Prado-Ribeiro, Thaís Bianca Brandão, Karina Morais Faria, Elisa Kauark Fontes, and Regina Maria Holanda de Mendonça

7 **Dysgeusia** 41
Natalia Rangel Palmier, Marcio Ajudarte Lopes, and Joel B. Epstein

8 Trismus 45
Ana Carolina Prado Ribeiro, Maria Cecília Querido de Oliveira, Thaís Bianca Brandão, and Luciana Estevam Simonato

9 Radiation Dermatitis 49
Ana Carolina Prado Ribeiro, Karina Morais Faria, Thaís Bianca Brandão, Rafael Tomaz Gomes, and Gustavo Nader Marta

10 Medication-Related Osteonecrosis of Jaws 55
Luiz Alcino Monteiro Gueiros, Letícia Lang, Camila Barcellos Calderipe, Caique Mariano Pedroso, Thaís Cristina Esteves-Pereira, and Marcio Ajudarte Lopes

11 Osteoradionecrosis 63
Luiz Alcino Monteiro Gueiros, Letícia Lang, Rogério de Andrade Elias, Maria Cecília Querido de Oliveira, and Aljomar José Vechiato Filho

12 Hyposalivation Induced by Radiotherapy 69
Luiz Alcino Monteiro Gueiros, Ana Carolina Prado Ribeiro, Marcio Ajudarte Lopes, and Regina Maria Holanda de Mendonça

13 Hyposalivation Induced by Graft Versus Host Disease 73
Aljomar José Vechiato Filho, Ana Carolina Prado Ribeiro, Maria Cecília Querido de Oliveira, Vinícius Rabelo Torregrossa, Thaís Bianca Brandão, and Joel B. Epstein

14 Antimicrobial Photodynamic Therapy in the Treatment of Osteonecrosis Related to Radiotherapy or Medication 77
Aljomar José Vechiato Filho, Maria Cecília Querido de Oliveira, Letícia Lang, Ana Carolina Prado-Ribeiro, and Luiz Alcino Monteiro Gueiros

Part III Oral Medicine

15 Recurrent Aphthous Stomatitis 85
Eliete Neves Silva Guerra, Juliana Amorim dos Santos, César Rivera, Karen Patricia Domínguez Gallagher, Eduardo David Piemonte, and Gloria Jeanethe Alvarez Gómez

16 Recurrent Herpes Labialis 89
Aljomar José Vechiato Filho, Maria Cecília Querido de Oliveira, Ana Carolina Prado Ribeiro, Diego Tetzner Fernandes, Leonor Victória González Pérez, and Márcio Diniz-Freitas

17 Lichen Planus 95
Rafael Tomaz Gomes, Luiz Alcino Monteiro Gueiros, Javier I. Giménez, Verónica E. Flück, Ángeles Castrillo, Claudia A. Giacco, Jairo Robledo-Sierra, and Joel B. Epstein

18 Pemphigus Vulgaris 99
Daniela Adorno Farias, Josefina Martínez-Ramírez, Wilfredo Alejandro González-Arriagada, and Pablo Agustin Vargas

19 Mucous Membrane Pemphigoid 103
Mariana Villarroel-Dorrego, Roberto Gerber-Mora, Vinicius Coelho Carrard, and Cristina Saldivia-Siracusa

20 Geographic Tongue 107
Lara Eunice Cândido Soares, Danielle Martins Startari, Ana Carolina Prado Ribeiro, and Juliana Lucena Schussel

21 Burning Mouth Syndrome 111
Thaís Cristina Esteves-Pereira, Ana Gabriela Costa Normando, Marcio Ajudarte Lopes, and Alan Roger Santos-Silva

22 Neuropathic Pain 117
Sven Eric Niklander, Markéta Janovská, and Arwa Mohammad Farag

23 Trigeminal Neuralgia 121
Manoela Carrera, Marco Antônio Trevizani Martins, and Manoela Domingues Martins

24 Facial Palsy 125
Arwa Mohammad Farag, Beatriz Nascimento Figueiredo Lebre Martins, and César Augusto Migliorati

25 Temporomandibular Dysfunction 129
Thaís Cristina Esteves-Pereira, Mariana de Pauli Paglioni, Francisco Javier Tejeda Nava, and Mario Nava-Villalba

Index 133

Part I
Photobiomodulation

The therapeutic use of light has its roots in antiquity, with sunlight being referenced in various scriptures. Furthermore, scientific evidence has demonstrated the efficacy of sunlight as a therapeutic approach for treating human disorders. In the latter half of the twentieth century, lasers were invented. Subsequently, a multitude of studies have been undertaken with the objective of elucidating the safety parameters, fundamental principles, and therapeutic outcomes associated with this approach.

Despite the existence of numerous terms that have been used to refer to the therapeutic use of light, including low-level laser therapy, phototherapy, and soft laser, a consensus was reached that "photobiomodulation" (PBM) is the nomenclature that should be used universally. PBM is defined as a form of light therapy that employs nonionizing forms of light sources, including lasers, light-emitting diodes, and broadband light within the visible and infrared spectrum. It is a nonthermal process involving endogenous chromophores that elicit photophysical (i.e., linear and nonlinear) and photochemical events at various biological scales. This process yields beneficial therapeutic outcomes, including but not limited to the alleviation of pain or inflammation, immunomodulation, and the promotion of wound healing and tissue regeneration.

Photobiomodulation therapy (PBMT) has emerged as a pivotal modality within the scope of practice of oral medicine specialists, offering a noninvasive, pain-free, and effective treatment option for a variety of oral conditions. Moreover, the potential for PBMT to influence the progression of chronic conditions extends beyond its role in symptom management. In oral medicine, where the preservation of function and quality of life is of paramount importance, PBMT offers a therapeutic avenue that not only addresses immediate clinical concerns but also supports long-term patient outcomes. As ongoing research continues to elucidate the underlying mechanisms and expand the indications for PBMT, its integration into oral medicine is poised to enhance patient care by providing a scientifically validated, clinically effective, and patient-friendly therapeutic option.

Further Reading

Anders JJ, Lanzafame RJ, Arany PR. Low-level light/laser therapy versus photobiomodulation therapy. Photomed Laser Surg. 2015 Apr;33(4):183–4.

Anders JJ, Arany PR, Baxter GD, Lanzafame RJ. Light-emitting diode therapy and low-level light therapy are photobiomodulation therapy. Photobiomodul Photomed Laser Surg. 2019 Feb;37(2):63–5.

Kauark-Fontes E, Migliorati CA, Epstein JB, Bensadoun RJ, Gueiros LAM, Carroll J, Ramalho LMP, Santos-Silva AR. Twenty-year analysis of photobiomodulation clinical studies for oral mucositis: a scoping review. Oral Surg Oral Med Oral Pathol Oral Radiol. 2023 May;135(5):626–41. Erratum in: Oral Surg Oral Med Oral Pathol Oral Radiol. 2023 Oct;136(4):529–530.

Mester A, Mester A. The history of photobiomodulation: Endre Mester (1903-1984). Photomed Laser Surg. 2017 Aug;35(8):393–4.

Chapter 1
Basic Principles of Physics in Photobiomodulation

Manoela Domingues Martins, Márcia Martins Marques, Thaís Cristina Esteves-Pereira, and Praveen R. Arany

Photobiomodulation (PBM) is a noninvasive therapeutic approach based on nonionizing sources of light, mostly lasers and LEDs, within the visible and infrared range of the electromagnetic spectrum (Fig. 1.1). The interaction of these wavelengths and biological tissues, in an appropriate combination of the laser system and the optical properties of the tissue, will result in beneficial therapeutical effects. The characteristics of the laser system are of importance in the laser–biological tissue interaction. On the other hand, the optical properties of the tissue involved in this interaction are refractive index, scattering coefficient, absorption coefficient, and anisotropy factor. PBM is a nonthermal therapy, which relies on endogenous light-absorbing molecules (chromophores and cytochromes) and light scattering within the tissues, triggering photophysical and photochemical reactions across various biological levels (Fig. 1.2). The overall results of these processes bring in the beneficial therapeutic effects mentioned above. Thus, PBM is an "adjunctive therapy" to be applied in practically all treatment procedures in dentistry aiming to improve the conventional treatments. Additionally, in some clinical scenarios, PBM may be used as a

M. D. Martins (✉)
Department of Oral Pathology, School of Dentistry, Federal University of Rio Grande do Sul, Porto Alegre, RS, Brazil

M. M. Marques
Department of Dentistry, School of Dentistry, University of São Paulo, São Paulo, SP, Brazil

University Ibirapuera Dental School, São Paulo, SP, Brazil

T. C. Esteves-Pereira
Oral Diagnosis Department, Piracicaba Dental School, University of Campinas, Piracicaba, SP, Brazil

P. R. Arany
Departments of Oral Biology and Biomedical Engineering, Schools of Dental Medicine, Engineering and Applied Sciences, State University of New York at Buffalo, Buffalo, NY, USA

A. R. Santos-Silva et al. (eds.), *Photobiomodulation Therapy in Oral Medicine*,
https://doi.org/10.1007/978-3-031-85048-6_1

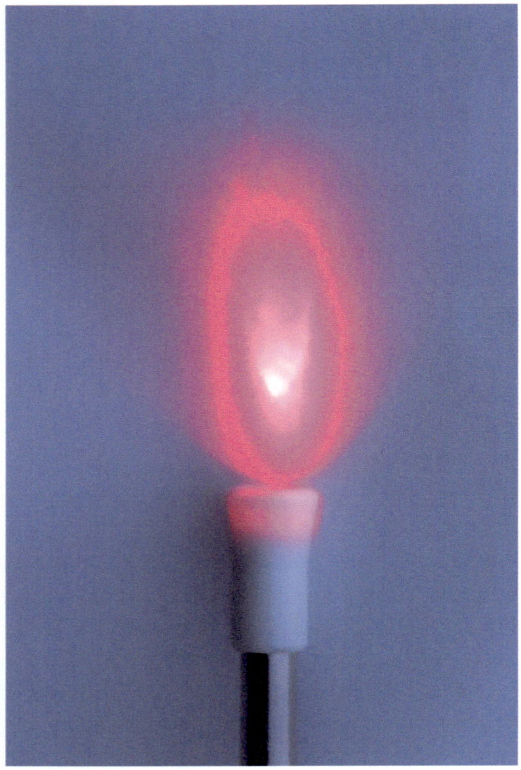

Fig. 1.1 Laser within the visible spectrum (red)

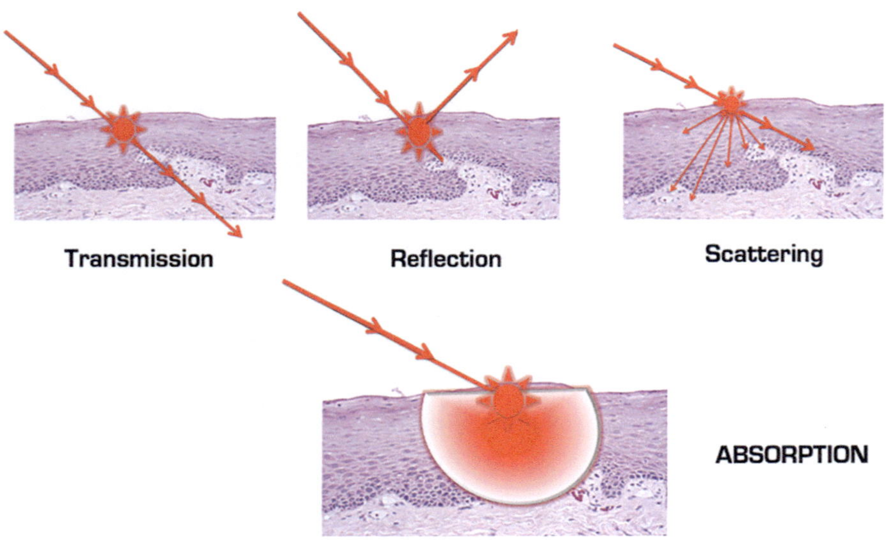

Fig. 1.2 Laser can have four types of interaction with the tissue, as follows: transmission, reflection, scattering, and absorption. It is dependent on the laser wavelength and the absorption characteristics of the tissue

mainstream choice of intervention such as in supportive cancer where the evidence for its role in management of oral mucositis is clearly established from human clinical trials.

As the reader will see in this book, the broad range of clinical applications of PBM is huge in dentistry and other health fields. The goals of photobiomodulation therapy (PBMT) are mostly control of pain and inflammatory process, immunomodulation, and tissue repair, by either wound healing or regeneration. Thus, PBM delivers pain relief by its analgesic and modulatory inflammation and immunology effects; moreover PBM promotes wound healing and tissue regeneration. These are the most expected effects to fulfill the needs of patients who are looking for treatment of several clinical conditions.

Endre Mester from Budapest in the later 1960s was the pioneer of the PBMT. And he already observed that PBM follows the Arndt-Schultz law or biphasic dose–response. This law is frequently invoked as an applicable theoretical framework for elucidating the dose-dependent nature of PBM effects. According to this law, the impact of stimuli on physiological activity follows a specific pattern: Weak stimuli augment activity, moderate stimuli suppress it, and exceedingly strong stimuli extinguish it altogether. Within the context of PBM, the escalating "stimulus" can manifest as an extended duration of irradiation or an elevation in beam intensity (measured in watts), total energy (measured in Joules), or energy density (measured in Joules per square centimeter or J/cm^2) delivered to the target tissue. PBM research has revealed a biphasic response, characterized by two distinct phases, although it necessitates evaluation across diverse tissue types, underlying pathological conditions, and PBM treatment protocols. Consequently, it is imperative to recognize that while this model aids in comprehending and investigating the role of dose rate, numerous other variables influence dosimetry in PBM, encompassing wavelength, tissue penetration depth, light attenuation, cellular target type, cellular condition, pulse patterns, and treatment intervals.

The clinical efficacy of PBM is contingent upon a constellation of parameters that can be broadly categorized into two major categories—device parameters and clinical delivery parameters. For the laser device, this includes wavelength (measured in nanometers), power density or irradiance (expressed in milliwatts per square centimeter or mW/cm^2), exposure duration (in seconds), fluence (in Joules per square centimeter or J/cm^2), total energy (fluence, measured in Joules or J), photonic fluence (includes wavelength energy, eV), and Einstein (photon Joules measured against 3 J/cm^2 at 810 nm, which is 4.5 p.J/cm^2). The mode of PBM devices can be continuous wave or pulsed, where the pulse duration, pulse energy, and repetition rate are critical. Prior reference to PBM, power output, beam spot size, and distance have now been combined into a single concept termed tissue surface irradiance that can be either measured or calculated. Treatment delivery parameters are a key component of PBM dose administration and can be either static, spot treatments, or scanning motion in either a raster, circular, or random pattern. Furthermore, other variables such as anatomical considerations, treatment site, clinical state, and individual subject characteristics can exert influence upon the clinical outcome.

The mechanisms underlying the actions of PBM, involving both lasers and LEDs, are now better understood. Numerous research investigations have been undertaken to shed light on the processes related to light absorption and the initiation of cellular signaling pathways. The effective tissue penetration of light and the specific wavelength of light absorbed by photoacceptors are two of the major parameters to be considered in light therapy. Upon illumination of biological tissue, light undergoes a series of interactions: Some is absorbed, some is reflected or scattered, and a fraction is transmitted through the tissue. Absorption is intricately linked to the transference of energy from the incident light to the tissue, instigating subsequent biochemical or biophysical alterations.

There is an "optical window" in tissue, where the effective tissue penetration of light is augmented. This optical window runs approximately from 400 nm to 1200 nm. Hence, the application of PBMT involves red to near-infrared (NIR) (600–1000 nm). Water and macromolecules, such as proteins and pigments, are responsible for absorption by biological tissues. It is foreseeable that besides proteins, the other three biological molecules, namely lipids, carbohydrates, and nucleic acids, could also be light modulated. This remains a ripe area of future research. The penetration of these wavelengths is then dependent of some factors, such as age and body weight, ethnicity, availability, health status, tissue, and location of the target tissue.

According to the First Law of Photochemistry, the photons of light must be absorbed by some molecular photoacceptors or chromophores for photochemistry to occur. Cytochromes are chromophores able to absorb low-power red and NIR light. Cytochrome c oxidase (Cox), the most known cytochrome, absorbs red and infrared light. However, other cytochromes are also relevant for PBM, such as calcium channels, cell membrane receptors, superoxide dismutase (Sod) enzyme, myoglobin, flavins, flavoproteins, and porphyrins. Once absorbed, light instigates a cascade of effects categorized as primary, secondary, and tertiary, ultimately culminating in biological responses.

Primary Effect

The primary effect of PBM is intimately connected to the depth of light penetration, a factor contingent upon wavelength, and the presence of chromophores. Within this primary effect, the most widely acknowledged molecular pathways governing PBM action are associated with the absorption of photons by chromophores found in the mitochondrial respiratory chain. Notably, the key chromophore in this context is Cox, a pivotal enzyme in mitochondrial complex IV within the electron transport chain, regulating mitochondrial respiration rate. The augmentation of Adenosine triphosphate (ATP) generation ensues because of metabolic processes initiated upon light absorption by the chromophore. This phenomenon predominantly occurs in cells in oxidative stress, wherein the presence of nitric oxide (NO) competitively binds to the heme-a3 and CuB centers of CCO, effectively obstructing oxygen (O2) and thereby interrupting the flow of hydrogen ions to the mitochondria

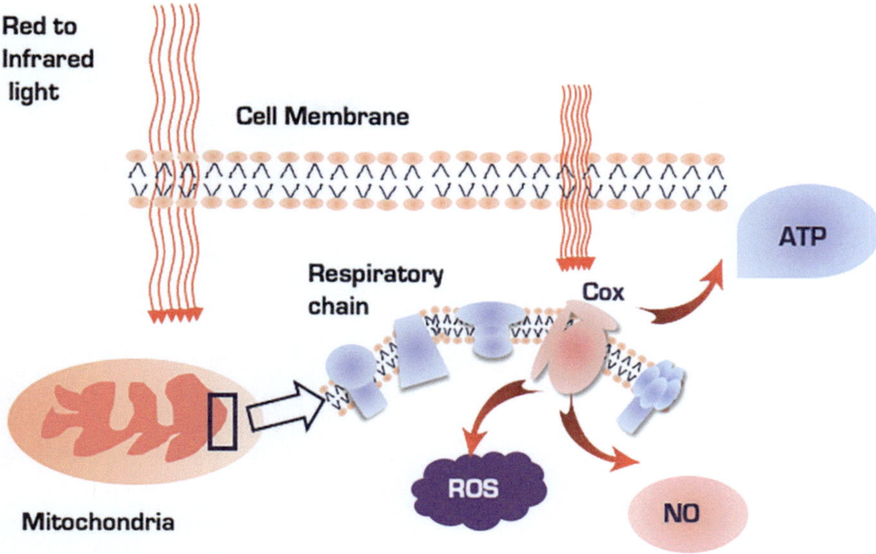

Fig. 1.3 The mechanisms underlying the action of red and infrared laser PBM involve the absorption of photons by Cox, a component of unit IV in the mitochondrial respiratory chain. This photon absorption results in the dissociation of inhibitory nitric oxide from Cox, thereby increasing enzyme activity and promoting heightened ATP production, accompanied by a surge in reactive oxygen species. The surplus ATP generated can subsequently activate the Na+/K+ ATPase pump

intermembranous space in the respiratory chain, which is responsible for ATP production. Upon exposure to radiation, cells experience the absorption of light by Cox, leading to the photodissociation of NO. This event triggers a transformation in enzymatic conformation, alteration of the redox state, modification of the rate of electron transfer along the respiratory chain, and activation of cellular respiration (Fig. 1.3). Consequently, this cascade results in the accumulation of reactive oxygen species (ROS), ATP or cAMP, and the modulation of NO levels.

Secondary Effect

The primary effects will culminate in the activation of transcription factors and signaling pathways, notably involving transcription factors, such as nuclear factor κB (NF-κB), Nrf-2, MAPK, PI3K, and JAK-STAT, among others. Moreover, the release of nitric oxide, a potent vasodilator, increases circulation, decreases inflammation, and improves the transport of oxygen and immune cells through tissue (Fig. 1.4). PBM can also exert influence on histone acetylation, thereby modulating chromatin accessibility and gene expression. These signaling pathways are widely recognized for their control over cellular processes including secretion, maturation, cell migration, and proliferation.

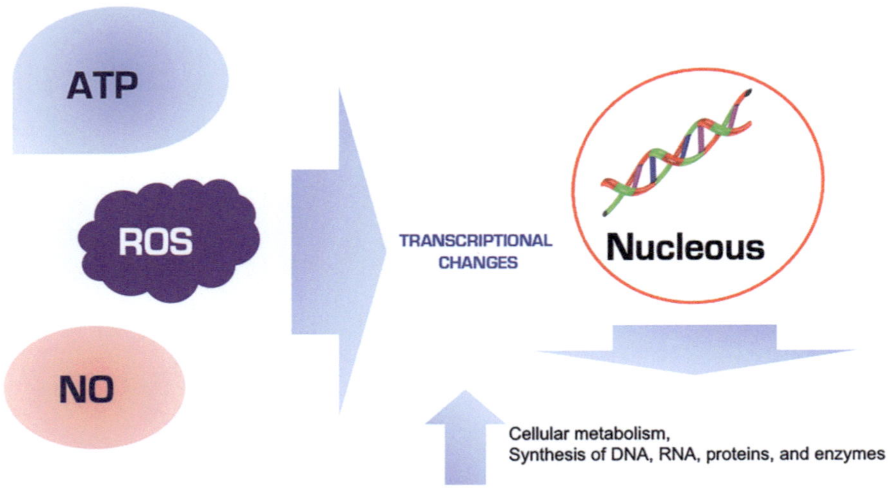

Fig. 1.4 The primary effects will culminate in the activation of transcription factors and signaling pathways that in turn will have effects on the cellular metabolism, increased synthesis of DNA, RNA, proteins, and enzymes within the nucleus and cytoplasm

Additional mechanisms involve the light-mediated modulation of cell membrane receptors, thereby influencing crucial ions like calcium (Ca2+), hydrogen ions (H+), and sodium/potassium (Na+/K+) transport between the intra- and extracellular milieu, significantly impacting cell physiology. This mechanism appears to be particularly relevant for the observed analgesic action and inflammation modulation associated with PBM. Another recently elucidated mechanism pertains to the activation of latent TGF-β1, a growth factor that exhibits diverse effects on various cell types of contingent upon the specific cellular context. Research has demonstrated that PBM induces the formation of ROS, subsequently altering the latent conformation of TGF-β and leading to its activation.

Hence, the primary effects transpire in the presence of light, wherein light absorption initiates biochemical reactions, subsequently giving rise to secondary effects. These secondary effects materialize independently of light and may manifest hours or even days following irradiation. They encompass heightened cellular metabolism, increased synthesis of DNA, RNA, proteins, and enzymes within the nucleus and cytoplasm.

Tertiary Effect

The tertiary effect on cells encompasses processes, such as cell proliferation, protein synthesis, cell differentiation, modification of nerve cell action potentials, impact on the immune system, angiogenesis, and modulation of cytokine and growth factor levels, among others. In the realm of tertiary effects, the response is intricately influenced by both internal and external environmental factors and intercellular interactions mediated by elevated cytokine or growth factor levels. These effects are well reported in the literature in in vitro and in vivo studies.

When it comes to the PBM in pain control, one can say that the mechanisms are complex and involve the blockage of nerve conduction. The suppression of neural activity also has the capacity to reduce inflammation by blocking the release of proinflammatory neuropeptides (substance P, bradykinin, and prostaglandin) from nerve endings. There is evidence suggesting that PBM therapy may cause: significant neuropharmacological effect on the synthesis, release, and metabolism of a range of neurochemicals, including serotonin and acetylcholine, at the central level and histamine and prostaglandin at the peripheral level. The pain influence has also been explained by the PBMT effect on enhanced synthesis of endorphin, decreased c-fiber activity, bradykinin, and altered pain threshold. Improving lymphatic flow is also an important component of pain relief. PBM promotes lymphogenesis, which increases the capacity to reduce swelling in long term.

Final Considerations

In general, the impact of PBM is typically ascribed to several key mechanisms, including the hastening of respiratory metabolism, a notable enhancement in mitochondrial membrane potential, and heightened mitochondrial respiration and ATP synthesis. These biochemical processes collectively lead to outcomes such as cell proliferation, prevention of cellular apoptosis, restoration of cellular metabolic functions, and the amelioration of pain and inflammation. There are many other proposals for mechanisms of PBM actions; however, one must have in mind that they are not isolate from each other, and probably they act together depending on the PBM parameters applied. More recently, there has been evidence that inelastic scattering may contribute to PBM therapeutic benefits, and this has opened new avenues to examine quantum effects within biological systems.

In conclusion, PBM offers significant therapeutic benefits to clinical dentistry and should be widely adopted. Paying attention to dose and mechanisms will enable for robust, reproducible clinical outcomes that can optimally benefit the patient.

Further Reading

Anders JJ, Lanzafame RJ, Arany PR. Low-level light/laser therapy versus photobiomodulation therapy. Photomed Laser Surg. 2015 Apr;33(4):183–4.

Arany PR, Cho A, Hunt TD, Sidhu G, Shin K, Hahm E, Huang GX, Weaver J, Chen AC, Padwa BL, Hamblin MR. Photoactivation of endogenous latent transforming growth factor–β1 directs dental stem cell differentiation for regeneration. Sci Transl Med. 2014;6(238):238ra69.

Arany PR, Nayak RS, Hallikerimath S, Limaye AM, Kale AD, Kondaiah P. Activation of latent TGF-beta1 by low-power laser in vitro correlates with increased TGF-beta1 levels in laser-enhanced oral wound healing. Wound Repair Regen. 2007 Nov–Dec;15(6):866–74.

Chung H, Dai T, Sharma SK, Huang YY, Carroll JD, Hamblin MR. The nuts and bolts of low-level laser (light) therapy. Ann Biomed Eng. 2012 Feb;40(2):516–33.

Cronshaw M, Parker S, Anagnostaki E, Mylona V, Lynch E, Grootveld M. Photobiomodulation dose parameters in dentistry: a systematic review and meta-analysis. Dent J (Basel). 2020 Oct 6;8(4):114.

Esteves-Pereira TC, Rawat N, Bensadoun RJ, Arany PR, Santos-Silva AR. How do clinicians prescribe photobiomodulation therapy (PBMT)? Harmonizing PBMT dosing with photonic fluence and Einstein. Oral Surg Oral Med Oral Pathol Oral Radiol. 2024 Dec;138(6):673–677.

Huang YY, Sharma SK, Carroll J, Hamblin MR. Biphasic dose response in low level light therapy – an update. Dose Response. 2011;9(4):602–18.

Mosca RC, Ong AA, Albasha O, Bass K, Arany P. Photobiomodulation therapy for wound care: a potent, noninvasive, photoceutical approach. Adv Skin Wound Care. 2019 Apr;32(4):157–67.

Parker S, Cronshaw M, Anagnostaki E, Mylona V, Lynch E, Grootveld M. Current concepts of laser-oral tissue interaction. Dent J (Basel). 2020 Jun 28;8(3):61.

Parker S, Cronshaw M, Grootveld M. Photobiomodulation delivery parameters in dentistry: an evidence-based approach. Photobiomodul Photomed Laser Surg. 2022 Jan;40(1):42–50.

Sommer AP, Pinheiro AL, Mester AR, Franke RP, Whelan HT. Biostimulatory windows in low-intensity laser activation: lasers, scanners, and NASA's light-emitting diode array system. J Clin Laser Med Surg. 2001 Feb;19(1):29–33.

Vladimirov YA, Osipov AN, Klebanov GI. Photobiological principles of therapeutic applications of laser radiation. Biochemistry (Mosc). 2004 Jan;69(1):81–90.

Wagner VP, Meurer L, Martins MA, Danilevicz CK, Magnusson AS, Marques MM, Filho MS, Squarize CH, Martins MD. Influence of different energy densities of laser phototherapy on oral wound healing. J Biomed Opt. 2013 Dec;18(12):128002.

Yadav A, Gupta A. Noninvasive red and near-infrared wavelength-induced photobiomodulation: promoting impaired cutaneous wound healing. Photodermatol Photoimmunol Photomed. 2017 Jan;33(1):4–13.

Young NC, Maximiano V, Arany PR. Thermodynamic basis for comparative photobiomodulation dosing with multiple wavelengths to direct odontoblast differentiation. J Biophotonics. 2022 Jun;15(6):e202100398.

Zezell DM, Ana PA. High power lasers and their interaction with biological tissues. In: de Freitas PM, Simões A, editors. Lasers in dentistry: guide for clinical practice. Wiley-Blackwell; 2015. p. 376. ISBN: 978-1-118-27502-3.

Chapter 2
Understanding Dosimetry in Photobiomodulation Therapy

Thaís Cristina Esteves-Pereira, Luiz Alcino Monteiro Gueiros, Praveen R. Arany, and Manoela Domingues Martins

Photobiomodulation (PBM) uses laser (high or low power) and/or LED in a non-thermal and non-ablative way. The widespread adoption of photobiomodulation therapy (PBMT) faces a significant obstacle because of nonuniformity in detail the dosimetry and clinical outcomes in several studies in the literature. Therefore, in this chapter, we will objectively address key parameters that should be collectivelly considered to understand the PBM protocol used and its effects, as well as the importance of their proper reporting in studies.

Drawing an analogy with medications, the PBM device functions like the medication itself, while the dose corresponds to how it is administered. Table 2.1 illustrates the main parameters and some brief explanation about them. Usually, for lasers fluence and energy are provided for each point irradiated, summing a total value depending on the number of points used. Irradiation parameters will therefore probably be crucial in determining whether results have a positive, zero, or negative impact. Consequently, it is crucial for PBM operators to comprehend these

T. C. Esteves-Pereira (✉)
Oral Diagnosis Department, Piracicaba Dental School, University of Campinas, Piracicaba, SP, Brazil

L. A. M. Gueiros
Clinical and Preventive Dentistry Department, Federal University of Pernambuco, Recife, PE, Brazil

P. R. Arany
Departments of Oral Biology and Biomedical Engineering, Schools of Dental Medicine, Engineering and Applied Sciences, State University of New York at Buffalo, Buffalo, NY, USA

M. D. Martins
Department of Oral Pathology, School of Dentistry, Federal University of Rio Grande do Sul, Porto Alegre, RS, Brazil

A. R. Santos-Silva et al. (eds.), *Photobiomodulation Therapy in Oral Medicine*,
https://doi.org/10.1007/978-3-031-85048-6_2

Table 2.1 Parameters for dosing photobiomodulation therapy in oral medicine

Device		
Parameter (unit)	Description	Observations
Wavelength (nm)	The distance between consecutive peaks (or troughs) of the electromagnetic wave represents one embodiment of the emitted light. In the analysis of laser light, the wavelength is the most fundamental property that determines the color or frequency of the laser light	The absorption of light is contingent upon the interaction between the wavelength and the various chromophores, which are endogenous compounds that absorb specific wavelengths. The shorter wavelengths are absorbed at the surface due to their interaction with melanin and hemoglobin. Longer wavelengths are capable of penetrating deeper due to their enhanced interaction with hemoglobin and water. Subsequently, the selection of the appropriate laser type/light based on its wavelength is of paramount importance to achieve optimal clinical outcomes
Output power (W)	This value represents the number of photons emitted from the device. This parameter is of great importance in laser systems, as it significantly influences the laser effect on tissue, particularly when considered in conjunction with the distribution over the treatment area (cm^2)	One of the most common methods of classifying lasers is by their output power, which is used to divide lasers into two categories: High-power lasers and low-power lasers. High-power lasers have a high energy absorption rate, resulting in a thermal effect. Low-power lasers have a low energy absorption rate, resulting in a nonthermal effect. PBM can be achieved with low-power lasers or high-power lasers in defocused conditions
Beam area (cm^2)	The term refers to the diameter of the laser beam, as measured at the exit face of the laser housing. This parameter is significant, as it affects the amount of effective energy delivered to the tissue	A larger spot size results in a more extensive distribution of energy over a larger area, which in turn leads to a reduction in the fluence. A reduction in the spot size results in a greater energy delivery to the targeted area, which in turn leads to an increase in the fluence
Dose prescription		
Energy (J)	Number of photons reaching the tissue per unit time	Energy (J) = power (W) × time (s)
Fluence (J/cm^2)	Energy density. The quantity of energy transferred to the tissue per unit area	Fluence (J/cm^2) = [power (W) × time (s)] / area (cm^2)
Irradiance (W/cm^2)	Power density. It represents the power of the laser that is distributed over an area. A notable alteration in the quantity of energy delivered to the tissue can be achieved by modifying the dimensions of the spot size	Irradiance (W/cm^2) = power (W) / area (cm^2) It has been demonstrated that lower irradiances (0.1 to 25 mW/cm^2) are optimal for wound healing applications. Conversely, higher peak irradiance (up to 150 mW/cm^2) has been shown to be most effective at relieving pain and inflammation

(continued)

Table 2.1 (continued)

Device		
Parameter (unit)	Description	Observations
Photonic fluence (p.J/cm^2 or Einstein)	Photonic fluence has been considered a more precise PBM dose concept as it considers irradiance, time and the individual wavelength-specific photonic energy	Photonic fluence (p.J/cm^2) = irradiance (W/cm^2) × time (s) × photonic energy (eV) 4.5 p.J/cm^2 = 1 Einstein
Irradiation time (s)	The time used can vary according to the equipment, power, fluence, or photonic fluence ideal for the condition to be treated	The reported variances in treatment time and number of spots appear to be poorly scientifically rationalized. Recent investigations suggested that a minimal treatment time and maximal irradiance that maintains a nonthermal (< 45 °C) tissue response should be used.
Form of application	Most PBM protocols require contact. Noncontact or defocused mode is used when high power is applied	The use of a PBM with a noncontact dose on the tissue surface and apparent volume underneath is more challenging to accurately control and report due to the potential for variations in manual scanning speed and the boundary extents of treated surfaces
Interval (hours, days, weeks)	In general, more than one session has been used to achieve optimal clinical outcomes	

parameters, receive appropriate training, and personalize treatments to effectively care for patients.

The numerous illness situations for which PBM efficacy has been established make it clear that a universal PBM dose is improbable. Besides that, approaching the dosimetry in PBMT might be challenging due to the difficult in understanding what is dose in PBMT. Is it radiant energy? Is it fluence? The traditional formula for calculating PBM dosimetry involves of modulating the irradiance, which is dependent on energy and beam area, and the exposure time. The product of these two variables gives the fluence value, measured in J/cm^2.

Currently, there are light source devices available with different wavelengths and power outputs. The use of multiple wavelengths allows for the direction of light at specific tissue chromophores, as the variation of wavelengths can be combined. These three points suggest that different biological responses can be achieved with multiple wavelengths, as the absorption of light by the chromophore is dependent on its affinity with the wavelength used.

By adding the photonic energy value that corresponds to the applied wavelength (Table 2.1) as a new variable to the traditional formula, a more precise dose may elicit a more predictable therapeutic response. This alternative paradigm for PBM dosing is called photonic fluence (Table 2.2).

Table 2.2 Wavelengths (nm) with corresponding photon energy values (eV)

Wavelength (nm)	Photonic energy (eV)
400	3.1
450	2.7
500	2.5
550	2.2
600	2.1
650	1.9
700	1.4
750	1.6
800	1.5
850	1.5
900	1.4
950	1.3
1000	1.2
1050	1.1
1100	1

Therefore, the initial step is to acquire the tissue surface irradiance by measuring it with a power meter. Equipment specification might provide this value. Next, the fluence is multiplied by the photonic energy value corresponding to the used wavelength.

$$\text{Photonic Fluence}\left(\text{p.J}/\text{cm}^2\right) = \text{Irradiance}\left(\text{W}/\text{cm}^2\right) \times \text{Time}\left(\text{s}\right) \times \text{Photonic Energy}\left(\text{eV}\right).$$

The term “Einstein” refers to the reference value of photonic fluence at 810 nm (1.5 eV) and 3 J/cm^2, which is 4.5 p.J/cm^2. To obtain the photonic fluence value in Einstein, divide the measured photonic fluence in p.J/cm^2 by 4.5.

$$\text{Photonic Fluence}\left(\text{Einstein}\right) = \frac{\text{Photonic fluence}\left(\text{p.J}/\text{cm2}\right)}{4.5}.$$

The aim of this dosing approach is to provide the most beneficial therapeutic dose to a target tissue, allowing certain individualized protocol parameters for the conditions managed and treated with PBMT.

At the end of each chapter of this book, the recommended protocols present the most detailed parameters possible. The beam area considered was 1 cm^2 for the purposes of convention, as this is a specific aspect of each device.

Further Reading

ADA Technical Report No. 189. Photobiomodulation (PBM) in oral health: the technology, science, and safety considerations. Standards Committee on Dental Products. 2023.

Chung H, Dai T, Sharma SK, Huang YY, Carroll JD, Hamblin MR. The nuts and bolts of low-level laser (light) therapy. Ann Biomed Eng. 2012 Feb;40(2):516–33.

Esteves-Pereira TC, Rawat N, Bensadoun RJ, Arany PR, Santos-Silva AR. How do clinicians prescribe photobiomodulation therapy (PBMT)? Harmonizing PBMT dosing with photonic fluence and Einstein. Oral Surg Oral Med Oral Pathol Oral Radiol. 2024;138(6):673–7.

Gobbo M, Merigo E, Arany PR, Bensadoun RJ, Santos-Silva AR, Gueiros LA, Ottaviani G. Quality assessment of PBM protocols for oral complications in head and neck cancer patients: part 1. Front Oral Health. 2022 Jul 7;3:945718.

Gobbo M, Arany PR, Merigo E, Bensadoun RJ, Santos-Silva AR, Gueiros LA, Ottaviani G. Quality assessment of PBM protocols for oral complications in head and neck cancer patients: part 2. Support Care Cancer. 2023 Apr 28;31(5):306.

Parker S, Cronshaw M, Grootveld M. Photobiomodulation delivery parameters in dentistry: an evidence-based approach. Photobiomodul Photomed Laser Surg. 2022 Jan;40(1):42–50.

Robijns J, Nair RG, Lodewijckx J, Arany P, Barasch A, Bjordal JM, Bossi P, Chilles A, Corby PM, Epstein JB, Elad S, Fekrazad R, Fregnani ER, Genot MT, Ibarra AMC, Hamblin MR, Heiskanen V, Hu K, Klastersky J, Lalla R, Latifian S, Maiya A, Mebis J, Migliorati CA, Milstein DMJ, Murphy B, Raber-Durlacher JE, Roseboom HJ, Sonis S, Treister N, Zadik Y, Bensadoun RJ. Photobiomodulation therapy in management of cancer therapy-induced side effects: WALT position paper 2022. Front Oncol. 2022 Aug 30;12:927685.

Young NC, Maximiano V, Arany PR. Thermodynamic basis for comparative photobiomodulation dosing with multiple wavelengths to direct odontoblast differentiation. J Biophotonics. 2022 Jun;15(6):e202100398.

Chapter 3
Equipment Quality Control and Selection

Thaís Cristina Esteves-Pereira, Wilfredo Alejandro González-Arriagada, and João Adolfo Costa Hanemann

Photobiomodulation (PBM) mechanisms focus on biostimulation and modulation at molecular, cellular, and tissue levels, offering therapeutic precision by targeting specific biological processes with light. Studies have shown that PBM can influence radiosensitivity and radioresistance of cells, affecting cell proliferation, colony formation, cell cycle phases, and cell death processes, highlighting the intricate ways in which PBM can interact with biological systems at various levels to promote therapeutic effects, as a promising approach for diverse medical applications. PBM utilizes a specific optical window for targeted therapy, with red light penetrating well suited for surface tissues, while near-infrared (NIR) light reaches deeper targets.

It is important for clinicians to note that PBM devices are subject to safety and reliability regulations and must be approved by local laws for both professional use and patient irradiation during equipment operation. These devices are used for various medical applications, including wound healing, pain management, and tissue repair. It is crucial for clinicians to adhere to these regulations to ensure the devices' effectiveness and safety for patients. Compliance with local laws and regulations guarantees that the devices meet specific standards, minimizing potential risks associated with their use in clinical settings. Therefore, clinicians should prioritize using approved and regulated PBM devices to provide optimal care while ensuring patient safety and treatment efficacy. However, PBM devices, including those utilizing light-emitting diodes (LEDs) and lasers, lack standardized regulations, posing

T. C. Esteves-Pereira
Oral Diagnosis Department, Piracicaba Dental School, University of Campinas, Piracicaba, SP, Brazil

W. A. González-Arriagada (✉)
Faculty of Dentistry, University of Los Andes, Santiago, Chile
e-mail: wgonzalez@uandes.cl

J. A. C. Hanemann
School of Dentistry, Federal University of Alfenas, Alfenas, MG, Brazil

A. R. Santos-Silva et al. (eds.), *Photobiomodulation Therapy in Oral Medicine*,
https://doi.org/10.1007/978-3-031-85048-6_3

challenges in assessing their safety and efficacy. While LED devices are cost-effective and do not require stringent laser safety measures, concerns exist regarding information bias and the absence of uniform protocols.

Therefore, professionals who handle the equipment for therapeutic purposes must have knowledge of equipment characteristics and parameters. When selecting a device for daily practice, the clinician should consider several specifications, including:

- Light source (laser or LEDs).
- Wavelength (red or NIR).
- Pulse frequency.
- Output power.
- Beam area.

Research has shown positive outcomes using both laser and LED devices as light sources for photobiomodulation therapy (PBMT). These devices, emitting wavelengths ranging from 618 to 1064 nm, have been utilized in various research studies. The efficacy of PBM has shown promising results in diverse treatments, modulating cellular processes effectively.

Research has shown that different output powers, ranging from 1 mW to 500 mW, can have varying effects on biological processes. The literature underscores the importance of selecting the appropriate output power in PBMT to achieve desired therapeutic outcomes in various applications.

The beam area of PBM has been extensively studied, showing that different handpieces used for PBM treatments can significantly affect the power density distribution, highlighting the importance of beam area optimization in PBM devices to enhance treatment outcomes and ensure consistent results.

It is important to note that there is a wide variety of devices available on the market. Table 3.1 shows the numerous PBMT devices used in the primary studies included in this book.

Table 3.1 Photobiomodulation therapy devices used in primary studies included in the preparation of this book[a]

Manufacturer (country)	Model (s)
A.R.C. Laser GmbH (Germany)	Fox
AixiZ Service & International, LLC (USA)	AH980-6015 AC
AMD Lasers, Inc. (USA)	Picasso Picasso Lite+ Picasso Lite 3.0
Asah Medico A/S (Denmark)	Unilaser 301P
Asalaser s.r.l. (Italy)	MLS® M6 MLS® MIX5
Atlantis Medical & Laser Equipment (Bulgaria)	SIX Laser TS
LLC Azor (Russia)	AZOR-2 K
Behsaz Gostar (Iran)	DLT 101
Bio-Art (Brazil)	Biolux laser

(continued)

Table 3.1 (continued)

Manufacturer (country)	Model (s)
Biolase, Inc. (USA)	Epic Ezlase 940 iLase LaserSmile Waterlase
Biophoton (manufacturer for triWings®) (France)	Travelers Oncolase®
Bioset Industry of Electronic Technology Ltd. (Brazil)	Physiolux Dual P.5040
Bison Medical Co. (South Korea)	Dental 5
Bredent Medical GmbH & Co (Helbo Medizintechnik) (Austria)	*NS*
BTL—Beautyline Technology Laser Ltd. (Czech Republic)	BTL 2000 therapeutic laser
BTL Medical International (Denmark)	BTL 5000
CB Medico (UK)	Master 3
Clean Line Industry and Commerce of Medical Dental Products Ltd. (Brazil)	Clean Line Easy Three Light
CMS Dental (Denmark)	DioBeam 830
Coherent Inc. (USA)	Compass-315 M-100
Cosmedical (Brazil)	Sportllux device
CTL—Centrum Technik Laserowej Laserinstruments Ltd. (Poland)	Doris, CTL 1106 MX
CuraLase (USA)	*NS*
DEKA M.E.L.A. s.r.l. (Italy)	Smarty A10
Dentoflex (Brazil)	Quasar VRkc-610 SOFT LASER
Dentsply Sirona (former Sirona Dental Systems) (USA)	SIROLaser SIROLaser Advance SIROLaser Xtend
DMC Equipments Ltd. (Brazil)	Flash Lase I Flash Lase III Laser Unit KM 3000 Photon Lase Photon Lase II Photon Lase III Thera Lase Therapy EC Therapy XT
DMT—Dental Medical Technologies s.r.l. (Italy)	DM980 RAFFAELLO 980 BIO
Doctor Smile of Lambda Scientifica s.r.l. (Italy)	Wiser
Ecco Fibras (Brazil)	Quantum
Elettronica Pagani (Italy)	Roland Serie CE Infrared-27
Elexxion AG (Germany)	Claros Pico
Eltech K-laser s.r.l. (Italy)	Arts Cube 4 K-laser Cube series K-Cube 3 K-1200-00149

(continued)

Table 3.1 (continued)

Manufacturer (country)	Model (s)
Enraf-Nonius (member of Zimmer Medical Group) (The Netherlands)	Endolaser 476
Eufoton (Italy)	LASEmaR® 800
Fisioline s.r.l. (Italy)	Lumix C.P.S. Dental Lumix 2
Fotona d.d. (Slovenia)	Fidelis Plus III Fotona XD-2
Fradama S.A. (Switzerland)	*NS*
Galbiati s.r.l. (Italy)	G-Laser 25
Garda Laser (Italy)	Ermes
GMT2000 s.r.l. (Italy)	Pointer Pulse
Good Energies Ltd. (Israel)	B-Cure Laser
Haemato (Poland)	Haemato LS PDT 660
Heltschl Medizintechnik GmbH (Austria)	ME-TL10000-SK
HTM Eletrônica (Brazil)	Fluence
IBRAMED® (Brazil)	Laserpulse Antares
Iranian Atomic Energy Agency (Iran)	IR-2000
Iskra Medical d.o.o. (Slovenia)	Medio LASER Combi
KLD – Biosystems Electronic Equipment Ltd. (Brazil)	Endophoton
Kondortech Equipamentos Odontológicos Ltd. (Brazil)	BioWave
Konftec Corporation (Taiwan)	Aculas-Am series
Kroman (Brazil)	Compacto KC 651 Laser KC 651
Laser Beam Industry LLC (Brazil)	IR30 MultiLaser
Laserdyne PTY LTD (Australia)	OMNILASE
Lasotronic AG (Switzerland)	Med 107
Lasotronix (Poland)	Smart M Smart M Pro
Light BioScience, LLC (USA)	GentleWaves
Lumenis Be Ltd. (Israel)	Opus 20
Lumenis, Inc. (USA)	*NS*
Lumileds Holding B.V. (USA)	Luxeon I Emitter
Lumina (Russia)	*NS*
Lutronic, Inc. (USA)	HEALITE II
MDT Bioelectronics (Switzerland)	MOLIMEDpen©
Mectronic Medicale s.r.l. (Italy)	iLux
Medic Tinedic (Denmark)	BTL 2000 Powerlase
MediCom (Czech Republic)	Maestro
Mediform (Spain)	Frank Line

(continued)

Table 3.1 (continued)

Manufacturer (country)	Model (s)
MMOptics Ltd. (Brazil)	Hand Duo Fisio LED Laser Duo Laser Hand Mucolaser Twin Laser Twin Flex Twin Flex II Twin Flex Evolution
NONO Enterprise Ltd. (Israel)	NONO 660
Optics Group of the Optics and Photonics Research Center (Physics Institute of São Carlos, University of São Paulo) (Brazil)	LASERTable
ORALIA medical GmbH (Germany)	Oralaser 1010 Oralaser Voxx
Oriel® Instruments (a Newport Corporation brand) (USA)	LTIO00-PLT20
PhotoMedex, Inc. (USA)	XTRAC laser AL 7000
PhotoTherapeutic (UK)	OmniLux Clar-U
Quantum Devices, Inc. (USA)	Spectralife
Quantum Láser Terapéutico (Laser Systems) (Mexico)	Quantum IR 810
Quantum Warp Light Devices (a division of JNME, LLC) (USA)	Quantum Warp 75
Rønvig Dental Mfg. A/S (Denmark)	Biophoton laser
Scientific-Research Center "Matrix" (Russia)	Matrix-2 k
SNJ Co., Ltd. (South Korea)	SNJ-1000
SpectraMedics Ltd. (Sweden)	Irradia™
Spectra-Physics, Inc. (USA)	*NS*
SPEX Forensics, Inc. (division of HORIBA Instruments Incorporated, a member of HORIBA Scientific) (USA)	Mini-CrimeScope MCS-400 SPEX
Syneron (Israel)	LiteTouch
TECE S.A. (Cuba)	Lasermed 670DL
Technika Ltd. (Russia)	Mustang Mustang 026 Mustang 2000 Mustang 2000+
Technoline (Serbia)	Medicolaser 637
Technomed Electronics (former Electro care Ltd.) (India)	Advanced Laser Therapy 1000 Laser 2001 Tech Laser SS-1000
Theralase Technologies (Canada)	TLC 5000
THOR Photomedicine Ltd. (UK)	DD2 Unit Lx2 Control Unit
Tianjin Lookout Photoelectric Technology Co., Ltd. (China)	*NS*
Union Medical Engineering Co. (South Korea)	UM-L25 special edition

(continued)

Table 3.1 (continued)

Manufacturer (country)	Model (s)
Weber Medical GmbH (Germany)	Weberneedle® Endolaser
WON Technology Co., Ltd. (South Korea)	*NS*
Wuhan GIGAA Optronics Technology Co. (China)	CHEESE
Zap Laser Ltd. (USA)	Soft Lase
Zolar Technology and Manufacturing Co., Inc. (Canada)	Photon

NS model not specified

[a]The data presented in this table were extracted from primary studies that reported sufficient information on the model and/or manufacturer of PBMT devices utilized in the protocols. Consequently, this table does not include all studies referenced throughout this book

The optimal equipment for a clinician is one that provides a satisfactory benefit-cost ratio in terms of safety, quality, and therapeutic parameters for clinical practice. It should also allow clinicians to adjust parameters to suit protocols for various conditions. Commercially available devices with predefined fluence and radiant values pose a challenge for research and clinical practice as they do not consider the individual characteristics of each subject and condition.

Preventive maintenance is necessary for quality control and expected therapeutic results in PBM equipment. Failure to perform routine maintenance can introduce significant uncertainty into the efficiency and effectiveness of PBMT due to discrepancies between manufacturer specifications and actual parameters.

Further Reading

Amaroli A, Arany P, Pasquale C, Benedicenti S, Bosco A, Ravera S. Improving consistency of photobiomodulation therapy: a novel flat-top beam hand-piece versus standard gaussian probes on mitochondrial activity. Int J Mol Sci. 2021 Jul 21;22(15):7788.

de Oliveira AR, Vanin AA, Tomazoni SS, Miranda EF, Albuquerque-Pontes GM, De Marchi T, Dos Santos Grandinetti V, de Paiva PRV, Imperatori TBG, de Carvalho PTC, Bjordal JM, Leal-Junior ECP. Pre-exercise infrared photobiomodulation therapy (810 nm) in skeletal muscle performance and postexercise recovery in humans: what is the optimal power output? Photomed Laser Surg. 2017 Nov;35(11):595–603.

Enwemeka CS. Intricacies of dose in laser phototherapy for tissue repair and pain relief. Photomed Laser Surg. 2009;27(3):387–93.

Girasol CE, Braz GA, Bachmann L, Celli J, Guirro RRJ. Laser light sources for photobiomodulation: the role of power and beam characterization in treatment accuracy and reliability. PLoS One. 2022 Mar 30;17(3):e0266193.

Glass GE. Photobiomodulation: a review of the molecular evidence for low level light therapy. J Plast Reconstr Aesthet Surg. 2021 May;74(5):1050–60.

Glass GE. Photobiomodulation: a systematic review of the oncologic safety of low-level light therapy for aesthetic skin rejuvenation. Aesthet Surg J. 2023 Apr 10;43(5):NP357–71.

Liebert A, Capon W, Pang V, Vila D, Bicknell B, McLachlan C, Kiat H. Photophysical mechanisms of photobiomodulation therapy as precision medicine. Biomedicines. 2023 Jan 17;11(2):237. https://doi.org/10.3390/biomedicines11020237.

Parker S, Cronshaw M, Anagnostaki E, Bordin-Aykroyd SR, Lynch E. Systematic review of delivery parameters used in dental photobiomodulation therapy. Photobiomodul Photomed Laser Surg. 2019 Dec;37(12):784–97.

Parker S, Cronshaw M, Grootveld M. Photobiomodulation delivery parameters in dentistry: an evidence-based approach. Photobiomodul Photomed Laser Surg. 2022 Jan;40(1):42–50.

Torres AE, Lim HW. Photobiomodulation for the management of hair loss. Photodermatol Photoimmunol Photomed. 2021 Mar;37(2):91–8.

Chapter 4
Cross-Infection Control in Photobiomodulation Therapy

Thaís Cristina Esteves-Pereira, João Adolfo Costa Hanemann, and René-Jean Bensadoun

Controlling infections in dental offices is a significant challenge for dentists, researchers, and immunologists. Microorganisms often circumvent safety measures, putting patients and professionals at risk. Dentists, like all healthcare professionals, must prioritize individual and collective protection methods.

The use of light therapy in medical and dental practices has become widespread in recent decades, and its benefits in dental practice are universally recognized. Therefore, it is necessary to adopt protective approaches that can prevent cross-infection when using this equipment in the dental office.

Cross-transmission of infectious diseases involves various factors, including microbial species, virulence, region, and frequency of exposure. Furthermore, the factors associated with the patient and oral healthcare practitioners can increase the risk of infection for both parties. They can act as hosts or reservoirs for pathogenic and nonpathogenic microorganisms.

Disposable barriers are marketed as a cost-effective way to avoid contamination of the light tip and prevent damage to the light guide caused by other factors, such as autoclaving, disinfection, and polishing procedures. However, it is important to carefully choose the biosafety material used as a protective barrier to avoid interfering with the therapy's outcome.

Photobiomodulation (PBM) equipment should deliver an appropriate dose to irradiated tissues. The amount and quality of irradiation, as well as the coverage area, affect how the tissue will respond to therapy. For all clinical indications of

T. C. Esteves-Pereira
Oral Diagnosis Department, Piracicaba Dental School, University of Campinas, Piracicaba, SP, Brazil

J. A. C. Hanemann (✉)
School of Dentistry, Federal University of Alfenas, Alfenas, MG, Brazil

R.-J. Bensadoun
Centre de Haute Energie (CHE), Nice, France

A. R. Santos-Silva et al. (eds.), *Photobiomodulation Therapy in Oral Medicine*, https://doi.org/10.1007/978-3-031-85048-6_4

Table 4.1 Disinfection and physical barrier protocol for photobiomodulation devices

Disinfection
Before each session, apply friction with a tissue soaked in ethylic alcohol 70%, for a period of 30 s
Physical barriers
Wrap the device and its probes in a disposable plastic film, such as polyvinyl chloride After the procedure, remove and dispose the plastic Repeat the disinfection with alcohol 70%
General recommendations
For goggles, use mechanical cleaning with water and soap The device and its probes should be manipulated wearing gloves. The pair of gloves used during disinfection is disposed, and a new pair is used for the procedure

PBM, there is a risk of cross-infection through direct contact of the equipment tip with the irradiated tissue. Therefore, it is necessary to protect the exit area of the laser that will meet the biological tissue by using plastic disposable barriers to prevent cross-infection.

The use of disposable plastic barriers is an affordable and noninvasive measure to prevent contact cross-contamination between oral tissues and the equipment used in dental offices, such as different light sources. The use of mechanical, disposable, and translucent barriers, such as polyethylene or polyvinyl chloride (PVC), has been proven to be an effective method of protection. Studies have shown that PVC is a suitable protection material for laser devices, regardless of the wavelength and equipment, as it is an accessible material that, when used correctly, can prevent cross-contamination without compromising the power output. Table 4.1 shows a protocol for disinfecting and protecting PBM equipment with physical barriers.

Further Reading

Arnabat-Dominguez J, Del Vecchio A, Todea C, Grzech-Lesniak K, Vescovi P, Romeo U, Nammour S. Laser dentistry in daily practice during the COVID-19 pandemic: benefits, risks and recommendations for safe treatments. Adv Clin Exp Med. 2021;30(2):119–25.

Besegato JF, Melo PBG, Tamae PE, Alves APAR, Rondón FF, Leanse LG, Anjos C, Casarin HH, Chinelatti MA, Faria G, Dai T, Bagnato VS, Rastelli ANS. How can biophotonics help dentistry to avoid or minimize cross infection by SARS-CoV-2? Photodiagnosis Photodyn Ther. 2022 Mar;37:102682.

Lago ADN, Cordon R, Gonçalves LM, Menezes CFS, Furtado GS, Rodrigues FCN, Marques DMC. How to use laser safely in times of COVID-19: systematic review. Spec Care Dentist. 2021;41(4):463–73.

McAndrew R, Lynch CD, Pavli M, Bannon A, Milward P. The effect of disposable infection control barriers and physical damage on the power output of light curing units and light curing tips. Br Dent J. 2011;210(8):E12.

Rodrigues FCN, Araújo JGL, Araújo EMS, Lago ADN, Mantilla TF, Freitas PM. Influence of biosafety materials of the laser output power. Lasers Med Sci. 2021;36(2):311–5.

Rodrigues JA, Hug I, Lussi A. The influence of PVC wrapping on the performance of two laser fluorescence devices on occlusal surfaces in vitro. Photomed Laser Surg. 2009;27(3):435–9.

Chapter 5
Safety and Adverse Effects in Photobiomodulation Therapy

Thaís Cristina Esteves-Pereira, Thaís Bianca Brandão, René-Jean Bensadoun, Elisa Kauark Fontes, Mariana de Pauli Paglioni, and Alan Roger Santos-Silva

When selecting a treatment, it is imperative that clinicians consider the evidence of efficacy and safety while balancing the risk and benefit for patients. Photobiomodulation (PBM) is a drug-free, safe, and cost-effective treatment modality that has demonstrated optimal clinical outcomes for cancer treatment toxicities and emerging evidence of efficacy in common oral diseases. Despite the promising clinical outcomes observed in oral medicine, the adverse effects of PBM are under-reported in the literature.

To date, no immediate adverse effects have been reported in the literature. Nevertheless, patients may experience numbness at the site of application and an increase in pain in the area immediately following photobiomodulation therapy (PBMT). These symptoms typically resolve within 24 h. Regarding delayed adverse effects or complications resulting from PBMT, there are no documented reports. The most frequently addressed potential late side effect of PBMT is its safety in malignant tumor sites, due to stimulating the growth of residual malignant cells that evaded oncologic treatment, leading to recurrences or the development of a second primary tumor.

T. C. Esteves-Pereira · M. de Pauli Paglioni · A. R. Santos-Silva
Oral Diagnosis Department, Piracicaba Dental School, University of Campinas, Piracicaba, SP, Brazil

T. B. Brandão
Dental Oncology Service, São Paulo State Cancer Institute, University of São Paulo Medical School, São Paulo, SP, Brazil

Oral Medicine Department, Sírio-Libanês Hospital, São Paulo, SP, Brazil

R.-J. Bensadoun (✉)
Centre de Haute Energie (CHE), Nice, France
e-mail: renejean.bensadoun@che-nice.com

E. K. Fontes
School of Dentistry, Federal University of Bahia, Salvador, BA, Brazil

A. R. Santos-Silva et al. (eds.), *Photobiomodulation Therapy in Oral Medicine*,
https://doi.org/10.1007/978-3-031-85048-6_5

A systematic review of 27 studies was conducted to evaluate the safety of PBMT use in the prevention and treatment of cancer-related toxicities. These toxicities included oral mucositis, lymphedema, radiodermatitis, and peripheral neuropathy. The findings of this systematic review indicate that PBMT is a well-tolerated treatment modality for cancer-related toxicities in the head and neck region, with no adverse side effects attributable to its use. The recurrence of tumors was not found to be higher or directly associated with the effects of lasers or LEDs.

A systematic review of 69 studies (in vitro, in vivo, and clinical with human subjects) revealed that the results were inconsistent across different study types. In vitro studies investigating the effect of PBMT on a diverse range of cancer cell lines have yielded conflicting results, which have been attributed to the parameters and frequency of PBM applications. Nevertheless, in vivo studies and clinical trials have demonstrated that PBMT does not induce tumor growth and may benefit patients by improving overall survival. They concluded that PBMT is a safe and effective treatment modality for the management of cancer-related side effects.

To mitigate potential risks, it is necessary to ascertain the clinical application of PBMT in each case and to delineate the intraoral spot location of application, particularly in instances of malignant tumors. Moreover, prior to initiating a PBM protocol, it is imperative to ensure that the patient is adequately informed of the potential benefits, risks, and alternative treatment options. During PBM sessions, it is imperative to adhere to appropriate biosafety measures (see the Cross-Infection Control in Photobiomodulation Therapy chapter). Additionally, clear guidelines for postprocedural care, including medication, diet, and oral hygiene, should be provided. Regular follow-up visits should be scheduled to monitor the patient's recovery and promptly identify any signs of complications.

Moreover, long-term follow-up clinical trials are necessary to ascertain the safety of PBMT in patients with cancer-related toxicities and those with common oral diseases.

Funding This work was funded by São Paulo Research Foundation (FAPESP)—grants 18/04657-8, 18/02233-6 and 18/234793.

Further Reading

Bensadoun RJ, Epstein JB, Nair RG, Barasch A, Raber-Durlacher JE, Migliorati C, Genot-Klastersky MT, Treister N, Arany P, Lodewijckx J, Robijns J. World Association for Laser Therapy (WALT). Safety and efficacy of photobiomodulation therapy in oncology: a systematic review. Cancer Med. 2020 Nov;9(22):8279–300.

Brandão TB, Morais-Faria K, Ribeiro ACP, Rivera C, Salvajoli JV, Lopes MA, Epstein JB, Arany PR, de Castro G Jr, Migliorati CA, Santos-Silva AR. Locally advanced oral squamous cell carcinoma patients treated with photobiomodulation for prevention of oral mucositis: retrospective outcomes and safety analyses. Support Care Cancer. 2018 Jul;26(7):2417–23.

de Pauli Paglioni M, Alves CGB, Fontes EK, Lopes MA, Ribeiro ACP, Brandão TB, Migliorati CA, Santos-Silva AR. Is photobiomodulation therapy effective in reducing pain caused by toxicities related to head and neck cancer treatment? A systematic review. Support Care Cancer. 2019 Nov;27(11):4043–54.

de Pauli Paglioni M, Araújo ALD, Arboleda LPA, Palmier NR, Fonsêca JM, Gomes-Silva W, Madrid-Troconis CC, Silveira FM, Martins MD, Faria KM, Ribeiro ACP, Brandão TB, Lopes MA, Leme AFP, Migliorati CA, Santos-Silva AR. Tumor safety and side effects of photobiomodulation therapy used for prevention and management of cancer treatment toxicities. A systematic review. Oral Oncol. 2019 Jun;93:21–8.

Kauark-Fontes E, Rodrigues-Oliveira L, Epstein JB, Faria KM, Araújo ALD, Gueiros LAM, Migliorati CA, Salloum RG, Burton P, Carroll J, Lopes MA, Alves CGB, Palmier NR, Prado-Ribeiro AC, Brandão TB, Santos-Silva AR. Cost-effectiveness of photobiomodulation therapy for the prevention and management of cancer treatment toxicities: a systematic review. Support Care Cancer. 2021 Jun;29(6):2875–84.

Pandeshwar P, Roa MD, Das R, Shastry SP, Kaul R, Srinivasreddy MB. Photobiomodulation in oral medicine: a review. J Investig Clin Dent. 2016 May;7(2):114–26.

Silveira FM, Paglioni MP, Marques MM, Santos-Silva AR, Migliorati CA, Arany P, Martins MD. Examining tumor modulating effects of photobiomodulation therapy on head and neck squamous cell carcinomas. Photochem Photobiol Sci. 2019 Jul 10;18(7):1621–37.

Silveira FM, Schmidt TR, Neumann B, Rosset C, Zanella VG, Maahs GS, Martins MAT, Arany P, Wagner VP, Lopes MA, Santos-Silva AR, Martins MD. Impact of photobiomodulation in a patient-derived xenograft model of oral squamous cell carcinoma. Oral Dis. 2023 Mar;29(2):547–56.

Part II
Supportive Care in Cancer

In 2022, oral cancer, a prevalent malignancy affecting the head and neck region, accounted for over 389,485 new diagnoses and resulted in more than 188,230 fatalities globally. Other areas, such as the oropharynx, nasopharynx, hypopharynx, and salivary glands, were responsible for over 368,000 new cases and approximately 190,555 deaths. Most patients typically present with advanced-stage disease, contributing to a poor prognosis, with an estimated 5-year overall survival rate of approximately 50%.

The management of advanced head and neck cancer (HNC) often necessitates multimodal treatment strategies, incorporating surgical interventions, radiotherapy, and chemotherapy. However, this comprehensive therapeutic approach is associated with considerable morbidity, encompassing both short-term and long-term sequelae. These ramifications can lead to functional impairments in critical aspects such as breathing, swallowing, and speech and may result in disfigurement.

Cancer is a complex and multifactorial disease, exerting a profound impact on both the physical status and psychological/relational dimensions of patients. Recognizing the intricate nature of this condition, the imperative for providing comprehensive information, counseling, and coordinated care by multiprofessional teams becomes evident. This approach holds promise in not only improving post-treatment outcomes but also optimizing the overall care performance in the treatment of HNC.

In addition to the direct collaboration between dentists and oncologists overseeing the patient's care, the integration of other healthcare professionals, including nutritionists and physiotherapists, assumes paramount importance. This collaborative synergy is indispensable, playing a crucial role in both the prevention and treatment of a myriad of alterations commonly encountered throughout the management of cancer-related issues. The interdisciplinary involvement of these healthcare professionals ensures a comprehensive approach to address the diverse physical, psychosocial, and nutritional needs of individuals undergoing cancer treatment, contributing to enhanced patient outcomes and well-being.

Further Reading

Bouvard V, Nethan ST, Singh D, Warnakulasuriya S, Mehrotra R, Chaturvedi AK, Chen TH, Ayo-Yusuf OA, Gupta PC, Kerr AR, Tilakaratne WM, Anantharaman D, Conway DI, Gillenwater A, Johnson NW, Kowalski LP, Leon ME, Mandrik O, Nagao T, Prasad VM, Ramadas K, Roitberg F, Saintigny P, Sankaranarayanan R, Santos-Silva AR, Sinha DN, Vatanasapt P, Zain RB, Lauby-Secretan B. IARC Perspective on oral cancer prevention. N Engl J Med. 2022 Nov 24;387(21):1999–2005.

Bray F, Laversanne M, Sung H, Ferlay J, Siegel RL, Soerjomataram I, Jemal A. Global cancer statistics 2022: GLOBOCAN estimates of incidence and mortality worldwide for 36 cancers in 185 countries. CA Cancer J Clin. 2024 May–Jun;74(3):229–63.

Gueiros LA, Gobbo M, Santos-Silva AR, Merigo E, Miranda-Silva W, Fregnani ER, Ottaviani G, Kauark-Fontes E, Bensadoun RJ, Arany P. Underexplored areas of photobiomodulation in oral oncology: an expert analysis. Photobiomodul Photomed Laser Surg. 2024 Oct;42(10):609–619.

International Agency for Research on Cancer (IARC) Oral cancer prevention. IARC Handb Cancer Prev. 2023;19:1–358. https://publications.iarc.who.int/617.

Schmid M, Giger R, Nisa L, Mueller SA, Schubert M, Schubert AD. Association of multiprofessional preoperative assessment and information for patients with head and neck cancer with postoperative outcomes. JAMA Otolaryngol Head Neck Surg. 2022 Mar 1;148(3):259–67.

Chapter 6
Oral Mucositis

Ana Carolina Prado-Ribeiro, Thaís Bianca Brandão, Karina Morais Faria, Elisa Kauark Fontes, and Regina Maria Holanda de Mendonça

Disease Definition

Mucositis can affect the gastrointestinal tract, from oral cavity to anus. Oral mucositis (OM) is a common consequence of chemotherapeutic infusion of stomatotoxic drugs or head and neck Radiotherapy (RT)—mainly for oral malignances—or the combination of both treatments. The early symptoms of OM are oral mucosal soreness or discomfort with red and smooth areas appearing in oral mucosa. In this stage, symptoms are normally mild (Fig. 6.1). When the integrity of the mucosa breaks down, ulcerations may occur in any site of the oral mucosa, although the nonkeratinized mucosa is more often affected (e.g., buccal mucosa, soft palate, and lateral border of the tongue and lips) (Fig. 6.1). In this moment, symptoms are more severe and challenging to manage. The grading scale of OM and consequently the severity of the condition can be classified according to Table 6.1.

It is often not possible to adequately assess the oral cavity in pediatric patients. In consideration of the morphological and functional aspects of oral mucosa, the

A. C. Prado-Ribeiro (✉) · K. M. Faria
Dental Oncology Service, São Paulo State Cancer Institute, University of São Paulo Medical School, São Paulo, SP, Brazil
e-mail: ana.prado@hc.fm.usp.br

T. B. Brandão
Dental Oncology Service, São Paulo State Cancer Institute, University of São Paulo Medical School, São Paulo, SP, Brazil

Oral Medicine Department, Sírio-Libanês Hospital, São Paulo, SP, Brazil

E. K. Fontes
School of Dentistry, Federal University of Bahia, Salvador, BA, Brazil

R. M. Holanda de Mendonça
Dentistry Department, Boldrini Children's Hospital, Campinas, SP, Brazil

A. R. Santos-Silva et al. (eds.), *Photobiomodulation Therapy in Oral Medicine*,
https://doi.org/10.1007/978-3-031-85048-6_6

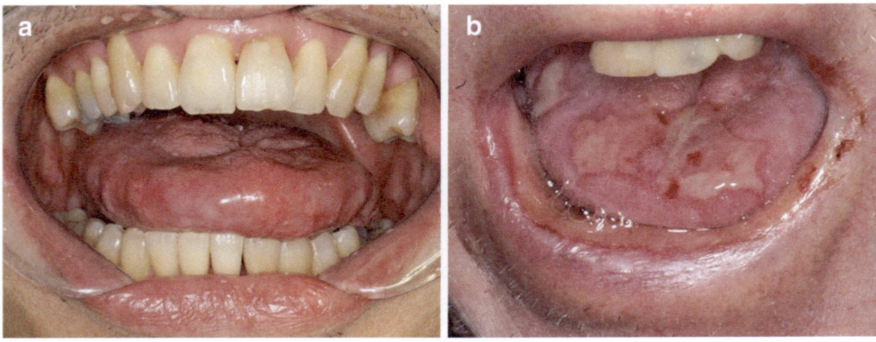

Fig. 6.1 (**a**) Tongue edema with red and smooth areas. (**b**) Ulcerations on the tongue and lower lips

Table 6.1 Grading scale of oral mucositis for clinical and research context[a]

	World Health Organization (WHO)	National Cancer Institute—Common Terminology Criteria for Adverse Events (NCI-CTCAE) v5.0
Grade	Description	
0	No oral mucositis	
1	Erythema and soreness	Asymptomatic or mild symptoms; intervention not indicated
2	Ulcers; able to eat solids	Moderate pain or ulcer that does not interfere with oral intake; modified diet indicated
3	Ulcers; requires liquid diet (due to mucositis)	Severe pain; interfering with oral intake
4	Ulcers; alimentation not possible (due to mucositis)	Life-threatening consequences; urgent intervention indicated
5		Death

For clinical use, the WHO scale is preferred. For research and clinical use with HNC patients, the NCI-CTCAE v5.0 is recommended

National Cancer Institute's Common Terminology Criteria for Adverse Events (NCI-CTCAE) v3.0 scale is recommended (Table 6.2).

In addition to the intense pain, OM increases consumption of opioids (narcotics), the need for nutrition support (nasoenteric and gastroenteric tubes and parenteral nutrition), risk of bacteremia, and extended hospital-based care need and may lead to discontinuation cancer therapy, which reduces the odds of long-term disease-free survival.

It is possible that individual features may increase the risk and progression of OM lesions. For instance, maxillectomized patients who use obturator prostheses may develop palatal mucositis at the interface of the prosthesis and the surgical

Table 6.2 National Cancer Institute's Common Terminology Criteria for Adverse Events (NCI-CTCAE) v3.0 scale for oral mucositis

Grade	Clinical exam	Functional/symptomatic
1	Erythema of the mucosa	Upper aerodigestive tract sites: minimal symptoms, normal diet; minimal respiratory symptoms but not interfering with function
2	Patchy ulcerations or pseudomembranes	Upper aerodigestive tract sites: symptomatic but can eat and swallow modified diet; respiratory symptoms interfering with function but not interfering with ADL[a]
3	Confluent ulcerations or pseudomembranes; bleeding with minor trauma	Upper aerodigestive tract sites: symptomatic and unable to adequately aliment or hydrate orally; respiratory symptoms interfering with ADL
4	Tissue necrosis; significant spontaneous bleeding; life-threatening consequences	Symptoms associated with life-threatening consequences
5	Death	Death

[a]*ADL* activities of daily living

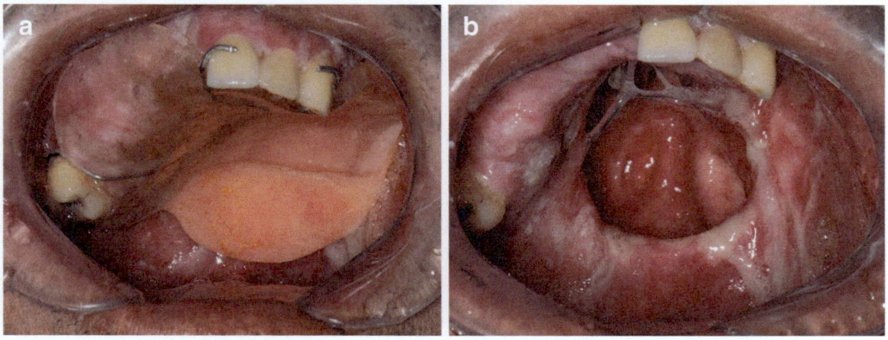

Fig. 6.2 (**a**) Irradiated maxillectomized patient using a maxillary obturator. (**b**) Palatal mucositis

defect very early on (Fig. 6.2). Patients who have undergone surgery may also develop mucositis at the graft site. Those with opportunistic infections, such as persistent candidiasis during treatment, experience worsening oral mucositis and typically require longer post-radiotherapy photobiomodulation (PBM). Palliative patients receiving hypofractionated radiation doses may also exhibit significant clinical deterioration in the final treatment fractions, as do patients with tumor necrosis (Fig. 6.3). Patients with OM present unique individual challenges and characteristics, making each patient distinct in terms of assessment and daily monitoring within these protocols.

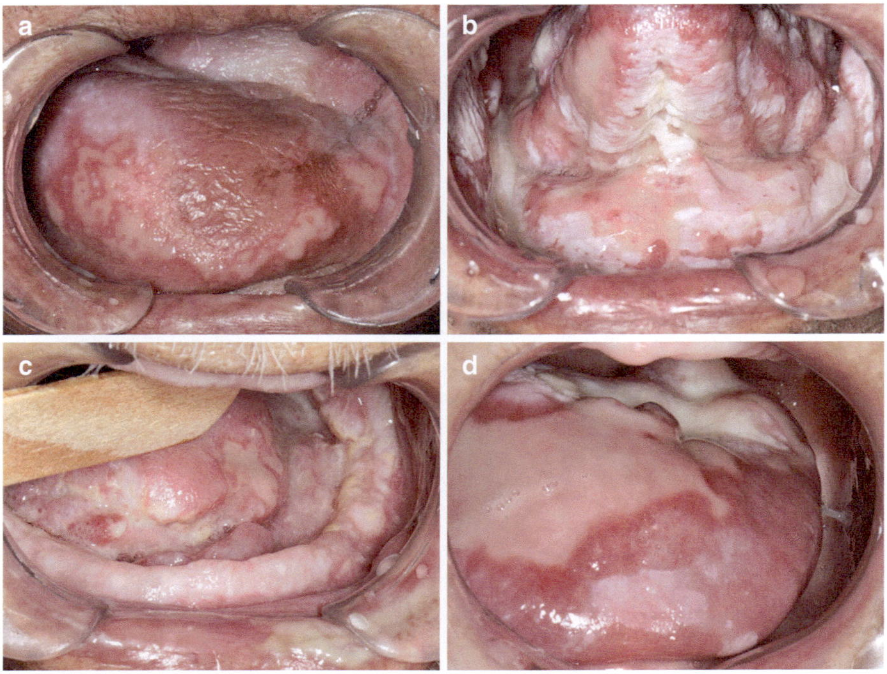

Fig. 6.3 (**a**) Irradiated patient presenting OM in floor of the mouth in flap area. (**b**) Irradiated patient presenting OM associated with fungal infection by *Candida* sp. (**c**) Irradiated patient present OM, tumor infection, and increased risk for bacteremia (**d**) Palliative irradiated patient presenting OM associated with extensive tumor necrosis in tongue

Diagnosis

- Clinical evaluation.
- RT in progress or recently finished irradiation.

Clinicians should consider other diagnosis hypotheses for OM-like lesions if ulcerations are still presented after 3 months of irradiation or more.

- Chemotherapy (CT) with stomatotoxic drugs in progress or recently finished infusion.

Clinicians should consider other diagnosis hypotheses for OM-like lesions if ulcerations are still presented after 2 months post-infusion.

- Hematopoietic stem cell transplantation (HSCT).

Clinicians should consider other diagnosis hypotheses for OM-like lesions if ulcerations are still presented after 2 months post-infusion.

Treatment

In 2020, the Multinational Association of Supportive Care in Cancer and International Society of Oral Oncology (MASCC/ISOO) updated its evidence-based clinical practice guidelines for mucositis. Treatment methods were categorized into seven groups: (1) basic oral care, (2) anti-inflammatory agents, (3) PBM, (4) cryotherapy, (5) antimicrobials, coating agents, anesthetics, and analgesics, (6) growth factors and cytokines, and (7) natural and miscellaneous agents.

PBM is a noninvasive and nonthermal technique used in the prevention and management of OM. The technique consists of an application of a high-density monochromatic narrowband light source, with various wavelengths in the visible red or NIR spectrum (632.8–970 nm).

In the prophylactic setting, PBM may delay the onset and decrease the severity of OM (mostly grades 1 and 2 of the WHO OM grading scale) and consequently prevent its more severe forms (grades 3 and 4), in which patient nutrition is significantly impaired, the use of opioids increases, and the risk of bacteremia is elevated. As a result, cancer treatment may be interrupted for symptoms control.

PBM can also be used in the treatment setting to enhance healing and reduce inflammation and pain by triggering a wide range of biological processes (Fig. 6.4). However, cells must receive an optimal dose of light for a better tissue stimulation and repair response (phenomenon is named as biphasic dose). Low levels of light have been associated with such desired tissue reaction than high levels, which may have an inhibitory effect. Table 6.3 displays PBM parameters for OM prevention and treatment.

One of the challenges for the universal acceptance of PBM use in cancer patients is whether there is a potential for the light to stimulate the growth of residual malignant cells that evaded oncologic treatment, increasing the risk for tumor recurrences and development of a second primary tumor. No clinical side effects have been reported. A systematic review conducted to check PBM safety suggests that the use of PBM therapy in the prevention and management of cancer treatment toxicities

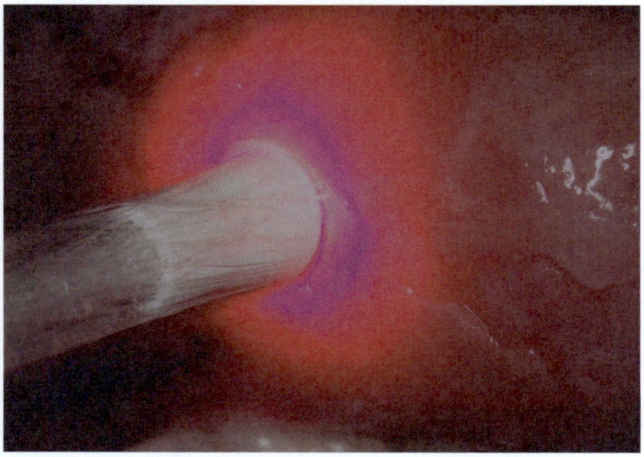

Fig. 6.4 PBM (660 nm laser) in OM on the tongue

Table 6.3 Photobiomodulation parameters suggested for preventing and treating oral mucositis

Wavelength (nm)		Red: 632.8–685	NIR: 780–830
Power (mW)		60–100	
Radiant energy (J)		≥ 1–2/point	
Fluence (J/cm²)		0.6–1.0	
Photonic fluence	(p.J/cm²)	≈ 1.1–1.2	≈ 0.9–1.6
	(Einstein)	≈ 0.2–0.4	≈ 0.2–0.3
Exposure time (s/point)		≥ 10–30	
Spot location		Prevention: entire accessible oral cavity (except at tumor lesion) Treatment: lesion (ulcerative or erythema)	
Treatment days		Prophylaxis: from the first day of RT/CT until the RT conclusion, until the first of CT[a] nadir[b] or HSCT engraftment Treatment: from the first day of lesion until complete healing or clinical improvement of the patient	

[a]Chemotherapy protocols with stomatotoxic drugs
[b]Lowest blood cell counts during each cycle of chemotherapy. It is assumed that the majority of drugs reach their nadir between 7 and 14 days post-infusion

does not lead to the development of tumor safety issues. This study included 152 oral squamous cell carcinoma (OSCC) patients and showed that the prophylactic use of PBM for OM did not impact treatment outcomes of the primary cancer, recurrence or new primary tumors, or survival in advanced OSCC patients.

Treatment

- *Systemic Pharmacological Treatment.*
  - Analgesics and anti-inflammatory drugs.

It is recommended to discuss with the patient's oncologist or radio-oncologist the prescription of opioids to ensure the most suitable analgesic protocol. Physicians usually consider all steps of pain management scale when prescribing analgesics.

- *Topical Pharmacological Treatment.*
  - Anti-inflammatory and analgesic mouth rinses (benzydamine mouthwash).
  - Anesthetics sprays (2% lidocaine gel or 10% lidocaine spray; the last suggestion is mostly available only for hospital facilities).

Given the difficulty children have in perceiving when they are anesthetized, which can lead to the risk of biting or aspiration of solid or liquid foods, it is recommended that its use be avoided in young children.

- *Miscellaneous.*
  - Maintenance of good oral hygiene (soft or extra soft bristle toothbrush and gentle, mild-tasting toothpaste with prescription-strength fluoride).

  - Cryotherapy (only for HSCT patients when CT protocol includes melphalan or 5-fluorouracil bolus).
- *Photobiomodulation.*

Funding This work was funded by São Paulo Research Foundation (FAPESP)—grants 16/22862-2, 18/02233-6 and 18/23479-3.

Further Reading

Brandão TB, Morais-Faria K, Ribeiro ACP, Rivera C, Salvajoli JV, Lopes MA, Epstein JB, Arany PR, de Castro G Jr, Migliorati CA, Santos-Silva AR. Locally advanced oral squamous cell carcinoma patients treated with photobiomodulation for prevention of oral mucositis: retrospective outcomes and safety analyses. Support Care Cancer. 2018 Jul;26(7):2417–23.

Cronshaw M, Parker S, Anagnostaki E, Mylona V, Lynch E, Grootveld M. Photobiomodulation and oral mucositis: a systematic review. Dent J (Basel). 2020 Aug 5;8(3):87.

de Pauli Paglioni M, Alves CGB, Fontes EK, Lopes MA, Ribeiro ACP, Brandão TB, Migliorati CA, Santos-Silva AR. Is photobiomodulation therapy effective in reducing pain caused by toxicities related to head and neck cancer treatment? A systematic review. Support Care Cancer. 2019 Nov;27(11):4043–54.

de Pauli Paglioni M, Araújo ALD, Arboleda LPA, Palmier NR, Fonsêca JM, Gomes-Silva W, Madrid-Troconis CC, Silveira FM, Martins MD, Faria KM, Ribeiro ACP, Brandão TB, Lopes MA, Leme AFP, Migliorati CA, Santos-Silva AR. Tumor safety and side effects of photobiomodulation therapy used for prevention and management of cancer treatment toxicities. A systematic review. Oral Oncol. 2019 Jun;93:21–8.

de Pauli Paglioni M, Faria KM, Palmier NR, Prado-Ribeiro AC, Edias RB, da Graça Pinto H, Treister NS, Epstein JB, Migliorati CA, Santos-Silva AR, Brandão TB. Patterns of oral mucositis in advanced oral squamous cell carcinoma patients managed with prophylactic photobiomodulation therapy-insights for future protocol development. Lasers Med Sci. 2021 Mar;36(2):429–36.

Elad S, Cheng KKF, Lalla RV, Yarom N, Hong C, Logan RM, Bowen J, Gibson R, Saunders DP, Zadik Y, Ariyawardana A, Correa ME, Ranna V, Bossi P. Mucositis Guidelines Leadership Group of the Multinational Association of Supportive Care in Cancer and International Society of Oral Oncology (MASCC/ISOO). MASCC/ISOO clinical practice guidelines for the management of mucositis secondary to cancer therapy. Cancer. 2020 Oct 1;126(19):4423–31. Erratum in: Cancer. 2021 Oct 1;127(19):3700.

Faria KM, Gomes-Silva W, Kauark-Fontes E, Bonfim-Alves CG, Kowalski LP, Prado-Ribeiro AC, Vechiato-Filho AJ, Lopes MA, Marta GN, de Castro G Jr, Leme AFP, Migliorati CA, Santos-Silva AR, Brandão TB. Impact of pandemic COVID-19 outbreak on oral mucositis preventive and treatment protocols: new perspectives for extraoral photobiomodulation therapy. Support Care Cancer. 2020 Oct;28(10):4545–8. Erratum in: Support Care Cancer. 2021 Jul;29(7):4177.

He M, Zhang B, Shen N, Wu N, Sun J. A systematic review and meta-analysis of the effect of low-level laser therapy (LLLT) on chemotherapy-induced oral mucositis in pediatric and young patients. Eur J Pediatr. 2018 Jan;177(1):7–17.

Kauark-Fontes E, Araújo ALD, Andrade DO, Faria KM, Prado-Ribeiro AC, Laheij A, Rios RA, Ramalho LMP, Brandão TB, Santos-Silva AR. Machine learning prediction model for oral mucositis risk in head and neck radiotherapy: a preliminary study. Support Care Cancer. 2025 Jan 14;33(2):96.

Kauark-Fontes E, Migliorati CA, Epstein JB, Bensadoun RJ, Gueiros LAM, Carroll J, Ramalho LMP, Santos-Silva AR. Twenty-year analysis of photobiomodulation clinical studies for oral mucositis: a scoping review. Oral Surg Oral Med Oral Pathol Oral Radiol. 2023 May;135(5):626–41 Erratum in: Oral Surg Oral Med Oral Pathol Oral Radiol. 2023 Oct;136(4):529–30.

Kauark-Fontes E, Migliorati CA, Epstein JB, Treister NS, Alves CGB, Faria KM, Palmier NR, Rodrigues-Oliveira L, de Pauli Paglioni M, Gueiros LAM, da Conceição Vasconcelos KGM, de Castro G Jr, Leme AFP, Lopes MA, Prado-Ribeiro AC, Brandão TB, Santos-Silva AR. Extraoral photobiomodulation for prevention of oral and oropharyngeal mucositis in head and neck cancer patients: interim analysis of a randomized, double-blind, clinical trial. Support Care Cancer. 2022 Mar;30(3):2225–36.

Legouté F, Bensadoun RJ, Seegers V, Pointreau Y, Caron D, Lang P, Prévost A, Martin L, Schick U, Morvant B, Capitain O, Calais G, Jadaud E. Low-level laser therapy in treatment of chemoradiotherapy-induced mucositis in head and neck cancer: results of a randomised, triple blind, multicentre phase III trial. Radiat Oncol. 2019 May 22;14(1):83.

Morais-Faria K, Palmier NR, de Lima Correia J, de Castro Júnior G, Dias RB, da Graça Pinto H, Lopes MA, Ribeiro ACP, Brandão TB, Santos-Silva AR. Young head and neck cancer patients are at increased risk of developing oral mucositis and trismus. Support Care Cancer. 2020 Sep;28(9):4345–52.

National Cancer Institute. Common Terminology Criteria for Adverse Events (CTCAE) Version 5.0 published: November 27, 2017. https://ctep.cancer.gov/protocoldevelopment/electronic_applications/docs/CTCAE_v5_Quick_Reference_5x7.pdf. Accessed 10 May 2024.

National Cancer Institute. Common Terminology Criteria for Adverse Events (CTCAE) Version 3.0. https://ctep.cancer.gov/protocolDevelopment/electronic_applications/docs/ctcaev3.pdf. Accessed 15 May 2024.

Potrich AR, Só BB, Schuch LF, Wagner VP, Silveira FM, de Abreu Alves F, Prado-Ribeiro AC, Santos-Silva AR, Treister NS, Martins MD, Martins MAT. Impact of photobiomodulation for prevention of oral mucositis on the quality of life of patients with head and neck cancer: a systematic review. Lasers Med Sci. 2023 Dec 7;39(1):1.

Zadik Y, Arany PR, Fregnani ER, Bossi P, Antunes HS, Bensadoun RJ, Gueiros LA, Majorana A, Nair RG, Ranna V, Tissing WJE, Vaddi A, Lubart R, Migliorati CA, Lalla RV, Cheng KKF, Elad S. Mucositis Study Group of the Multinational Association of Supportive Care in Cancer/International Society of Oral Oncology (MASCC/ISOO). Systematic review of photobiomodulation for the management of oral mucositis in cancer patients and clinical practice guidelines. Support Care Cancer. 2019 Oct;27(10):3969–83.

Chapter 7
Dysgeusia

Natalia Rangel Palmier, Marcio Ajudarte Lopes, and Joel B. Epstein

Disease Definition

Dysgeusia (or also described in literature as "altered taste perception") encompasses a myriad of taste alterations that range from diminished taste acuity, aversive taste sensations that can evolve to an extreme total loss of gustatory perception. The sensation of taste and flavor is a complex phenomenon that is influenced by a multitude of factors, including olfactory perception, salivation, infection, dietary intake, and local oral conditions. In addition, the temperature, texture, and appearance of food also influence taste perception. Injury to the afferent nerves that supply taste bud cells, head and neck trauma or surgery, infections, radiotherapy, chemotherapy, targeted therapy, and immune checkpoint inhibitors may be contributing factors.

Literature shows that dysgeusia is one of the most frequent side effects in patients undergoing chemotherapy (CT) protocols including cisplatin, 5-fluorouracil, and taxanes which have been associated with a direct effect on taste bud cell proliferation. Taste alteration has been reported by patients undergoing different oncologic treatment protocols. Studies have indicated that over 95% of patients submitted to head and neck

N. R. Palmier
Dental Oncology Service, São Paulo State Cancer Institute, University of São Paulo Medical School, São Paulo, SP, Brazil

Oral Medicine Department, Sírio-Libanês Hospital, São Paulo, SP, Brazil

M. A. Lopes (✉)
Oral Diagnosis Department, Piracicaba Dental School, University of Campinas, Piracicaba, SP, Brazil
e-mail: malopes@fop.unicamp.br

J. B. Epstein
Cedars-Sinai Health System, Los Angeles, CA, USA

City of Hope National Medical Center, Duarte, CA, USA

A. R. Santos-Silva et al. (eds.), *Photobiomodulation Therapy in Oral Medicine*,
https://doi.org/10.1007/978-3-031-85048-6_7

radiotherapy suffer from this toxicity. Such undesired complication has shown the same pattern in patients submitted to hematopoietic stem cell transplantation, as well. Usually, patients affected by this condition report a bitter, metallic, salty, and/or unpleasant taste during the course and even months after the oncologic treatment.

Dysgeusia is a matter of concern because change in taste or its total absence may lead to reduced food intake as patients do not feel pleasure during feeding, leading to malnutrition and cachexia and need for nasogastric tube feeding. Therefore, cancer treatment interruptions may occur, potentially requiring hospitalizations and leading to a decline in patients' quality of life.

The exact mechanism underlying the taste dysfunction in cancer patients is yet unknown. It is suggested that the destruction taste and olfactory receptor cells cause the disturbance in taste perception, and several mechanisms have been associated with the onset of dysgeusia in oncologic patients such as direct radiogenic effect, irradiated volume of the tongue specially its anterior portion, and damage to neural structures. Current literature includes studies with heterogeneous cancer populations, with a wide range of symptoms, and with lack of correlation with specific biologic markers.

Diagnosis

- Clinical evaluation.
- Taste testing.

Clinical evaluation with target questions is the easiest method for dysgeusia diagnosis, and the National Cancer Institute's Common Terminology Criteria for Adverse Events (NCI-CTCAE) v5.0 is one of the most used grading systems although it does not quantify the different alterations in flavor perception.

- Taste testing.

Chemical tests can assess patients' taste recognition by exposing them to different concentrations of substances representing each of the five known flavors: sweet, sour, salty, bitter, and umami. These tests are typically conducted as the whole mouth test, the taste strips test, and the filter paper test.

- Electrogustometry (EGM) test.

EGM test may also be applied in clinical settings to assess the tongue gustatory response to electrical stimulation.

Treatment

Up to date no clinically validated methods have been stablished for the treatment of dysgeusia. Dysgeusia management has been an important issue for oncologic patients; however, after the COVID-19 pandemic, more research has been carried

Table 7.1 Photobiomodulation parameters suggested for treating dysgeusia

Wavelength (nm)		Red: 635–660	NIR: 808
Power (mW)		100	
Radiant energy (J)		2–3/point	
Fluence (J/cm^2)		3	
Photonic fluence	($p.J/cm^2$)	≈ 5.7–6.3	≈ 4.5
	(Einstein)	≈ 1.2–1.4	≈ 1
Exposure time (s/point)		30	
Spot location		Ten points on the dorsum of the tongue; three points on the right lateral; three points on the left lateral	
Treatment days		Five consecutive daily sessions with 48 h of interval[a]	

[a]Consider repeating until positive response since there is no scientific evidence contraindicating PBM continuity

out with the aim of proposing an appropriate treatment for this condition. Literature shows a myriad of management techniques for dysgeusia such as zinc supplementation, photobiomodulation (PBM), acupuncture, herbal mouth washes, use of salivary substitutes, corticosteroids, ganglion block with local anesthesia, and curcuminoids, among several others, but so far none have been validated as a gold standard treatment protocol.

Although studies regarding the effectiveness of photobiomodulation therapy (PBMT) in treating dysgeusia are still scarce, a recent randomized and controlled clinical trial for treatment/prevention for CT-induced dysgeusia showed that PBM leads to a significant increase in body mass index, which may be associated with the low incidence of dysgeusia during treatment. However, the biological mechanisms explaining how PBM may benefit dysgeusia patients are not clear, as it was a reported unexpected clinical finding. Table 7.1 displays the suggested PBM parameters for dysgeusia.

Treatment

- *Systemic Pharmacological Treatment.*
  - Zinc supplementation.
- *Topical Pharmacological Treatment.*
  - Corticosteroids.
  - Saliva substitutes.
- *Miscellaneous.*
  - Herbal mouthwash.
  - Acupuncture.
  - Ganglion block with local anesthesia.
- *Photobiomodulation.*

Funding This work was funded by São Paulo Research Foundation (FAPESP)—grant 16/22862-2.

Further Reading

Blijleven EE, Wegner I, Stokroos RJ, Thomeer HGXM. The impact of injury of the chorda tympani nerve during primary stapes surgery or cochlear implantation on taste function, quality of life and food preferences: a study protocol for a double-blind prospective prognostic association study. PLoS One. 2023 May 18;18(5):e0284571.

Deshpande TS, Blanchard P, Wang L, Foote RL, Zhang X, Frank SJ. Radiation-related alterations of taste function in patients with head and neck cancer: a systematic review. Curr Treat Options in Oncol. 2018;19:72.

El Mobadder M, Farhat F, El Mobadder W, Nammour S. Photobiomodulation therapy in the treatment of oral mucositis, dysphagia, oral dryness, taste alteration, and burning mouth sensation due to cancer therapy: a case series. Int J Environ Res Public Health. 2019 Nov 15;16(22):4505.

Ha JG, Kim BR, Cho A, Jeong Y, Rha MS, Kang JW, Cho HJ, Yoon JH, Kim CH. Visualization of the relationship between electrogustometry and whole mouth test using multidimensional scaling. Sci Rep. 2023 May 31;13(1):8798.

Malta CEN, Carlos ACAM, de Alencar MCM, Alves E, Silva EF, Nogueira VBC, Alves APNN, Chaves FF, de Moura JFB, de Barros Silva PG. Photobiomodulation therapy prevents dysgeusia chemotherapy induced in breast cancer women treated with doxorubicin plus cyclophosphamide: a triple-blinded, randomized, placebo-controlled clinical trial. Support Care Cancer. 2022 Mar;30(3):2569–80.

Mazzoleni B, Ferrari G, Savioni F, Gravante F, Lopane D, Dacomi A, Coldani C, Tomaiuolo G, Cattani D, Anastasi G, Mancin S. Non-pharmacological strategies to alleviate dysgeusia in patients undergoing chemotherapy: a systematic review. Eur J Oncol Nurs. 2024 Mar 26;70:102569.

Mueller C, Kallert S, Renner B, Stiassny K, Temmel AF, Hummel T, Kobal G. Quantitative assessment of gustatory function in a clinical context using impregnated "taste strips". Rhinology. 2003 Mar;41(1):2–6.

National Cancer Institute. Common Terminology Criteria for Adverse Events (CTCAE) Version 5.0 published: November 27, 2017. https://ctep.cancer.gov/protocoldevelopment/electronic_applications/docs/CTCAE_v5_Quick_Reference_5x7.pdf. Accessed 10 May 2024.

Palmier NR, Mariz BALA, Rodrigues-Olieveira L, Morais-Faria K, Migliorati CA, Kowalski LP, Moutinho K, Brandão TB, Santos-Silva AR, Prado-Ribeio AC. Natural history of radiotherapy-induced dysgeusia among oral and oropharyngeal cancer patients undergoing different treatment modalities. Oral Oncol Rep. 2024 Mar;9:100185.

Parreira LFS, Pinheiro SL, Fontana CE. Photobiomodulation in the treatment of dysgeusia in patients with long COVID: a single-blind, randomized controlled trial. Photobiomodul Photomed Laser Surg. 2024 Mar;42(3):215–24.

Tsuruoka S, Wakaumi M, Araki N, Ioka T, Sugimoto K, Fujimura A. Comparative study of taste disturbance by losartan and perindopril in healthy volunteers. J Clin Pharmacol. 2005 Nov;45(11):1319–23.

Yamauchi Y, Endo S, Sakai F, Yoshimura I. A new whole-mouth gustatory test procedure. 1. Thresholds and principal components analysis in healthy men and women. Acta Otolaryngol Suppl. 2002;546:39–48.

Chapter 8
Trismus

Ana Carolina Prado Ribeiro, Maria Cecília Querido de Oliveira, Thaís Bianca Brandão, and Luciana Estevam Simonato

Disease Definition

Trismus is defined as limited mouth opening that may be associated with pain. It is one of the most frequent complications of head and neck cancer therapy, occurring between 5% and 38% of patients treated with extensive surgery and adjuvant radiation or exclusive radiotherapy (RT). It usually occurs 3–6 months after RT is completed with the potential to increase its severity up to 2 years. A restriction of the mouth opening of <35 mm is a well-supported cutoff point for trismus. Trismus can be developed after surgical procedures of malignant tumors because of scar formation in the muscles of mastication that limits mouth opening. It can also affect patients treated with RT of the head and neck area due to muscle fibrosis of the temporomandibular joint or of the muscles of mastication. The risk of developing trismus increases when the medial pterygoid muscle is included in surgical field or in the radiation areas.

Trismus can lead to difficulty in biting, chewing, and speaking, which negatively affects patient's quality of life. It may also impair oral hygiene, increasing the risk for dental caries and periodontal disease. Furthermore, trismus may difficult periodontal, restorative, surgical, and rehabilitation procedures and other dental treatments due to the lack of space for handling by professionals.

A. C. P. Ribeiro · M. C. Q. de Oliveira
Dental Oncology Service, São Paulo State Cancer Institute, University of São Paulo Medical School, São Paulo, SP, Brazil

T. B. Brandão
Dental Oncology Service, São Paulo State Cancer Institute, University of São Paulo Medical School, São Paulo, SP, Brazil

Oral Medicine Department, Sírio-Libanês Hospital, São Paulo, SP, Brazil

L. E. Simonato (✉)
Dental School, Brazil University, Fernandópolis, SP, Brazil
e-mail: luciana.simonato@universidadebrasil.edu.br

A. R. Santos-Silva et al. (eds.), *Photobiomodulation Therapy in Oral Medicine*,
https://doi.org/10.1007/978-3-031-85048-6_8

Diagnosis

- Clinical evaluation

Treatment

To date, several medical devices have been designed to assist in the rehabilitation of trismus. Exercise therapies with trismus devices (such as stacked wooden tongue depressors) are often prescribed, using stretching techniques to increase the range of mouth opening.

Photobiomodulation (PBM) has shown satisfactory results, being a contemporary and effective alternative for the treatment of trismus after RT. Some studies show positive clinical response obtained by the laser in its infrared spectrum (808 nm), through the PBM of pain in the trismus post-RT process (Table 8.1). The sensation of muscle relaxation and the improvements in muscle sensibility assessed through the Visual Analog Scale were reported in these patients included in those studies.

In therapy-resistant cases, trismus can be resolved by surgical procedures, generally performed by head and neck surgeons. However, the authors in the present chapter suggest to readership that trismus may be a symptom for tumor recurrence, and it should be investigated as its severity increases overtime, mainly in patients with maxillary tumors submitted to surgery and adjuvant RT.

Table 8.1 Photobiomodulation parameters suggested for treating trismus

Wavelength (nm)		NIR: 810
Power (mW)		100
Radiant energy (J)		3/point
Fluence (J/cm^2)		3
Photonic fluence	($p.J/cm^2$)	≈ 4.5
	(Einstein)	≈ 1
Exposure time (s/point)		30
Spot location		Extraoral: upper, posterior, and anterior points to the mandibular condyle and at an intra-auricular point toward the tragus Intrabuccal: one point bilateral located behind the retromolar trigone point
Treatment days		Ten sessions, twice a week for 5 weeks

It is important to observe if PBM applications are promoting positive results in trismus treatment. Therefore, surgical treatment may be considered, and PBM may be associated with enhance the postoperatory recovery

Treatment

- *Systemic Pharmacological Treatment*
  - Opioid analgesics

It is recommended to discuss with the patient's head and neck surgeon, radio-oncologist, or palliative doctor the prescription of opioids to ensure the most suitable analgesic protocol. Physicians usually consider all steps of pain management scale when prescribing analgesics.

- *Surgical Treatment*
  - Surgical treatment will be defined by head and neck surgeon.
- *Exercise Therapy*
  - TheraBite ® Jaw Motion Rehabilitation System

According to the expertise of the authors in the present chapter, using stacked wooden tongue depressors is the most effective and low-cost physiotherapy capable to improved mouth opening dimensions.

- *Botulinum Toxin Injection*
- *Photobiomodulation*

Funding This work was funded by São Paulo Research Foundation (FAPESP)—grants 16/22862-2 and 12/06138-1.

Further Reading

Borges MMF, Malta CEN, Carlos ACAM, Crispim AA, de Moura JFB, Rebouças LM, Coelho da Silva BC, de Albuquerque CGP, de Barros Silva PG. Photobiomodulation therapy in the treatment of radiotherapy-related trismus of the head and neck. Lasers Med Sci. 2023 Nov 8;38(1):259.

Charters E, Dunn M, Cheng K, Aung V, Mukherjee P, Froggatt C, Dusseldorp JR, Clark JR. Trismus therapy devices: a systematic review. Oral Oncol. 2022 Mar;126:105728.

Faravel K, Jarlier M, Senesse P, Huteau ME, Janiszewski C, Stoebner A, Boisselier P. Trismus occurrence and link with radiotherapy doses in head and neck cancer patients treated with chemoradiotherapy. Integr Cancer Ther. 2023 Jan-Dec;22:15347354221147283.

Hartl DM, Cohen M, Juliéron M, Marandas P, Janot F, Bourhis J. Botulinum toxin for radiation-induced facial pain and trismus. Otolaryngol Head Neck Surg. 2008 Apr;138(4):459–63.

Sollecito TP, Helgeson ES, Lalla RV, Treister NS, Schmidt BL, Patton LL, Lin A, Brennan MT. Reduced mouth opening in patients with head and neck cancer treated with radiation therapy: an analysis of the Clinical Registry of Dental Outcomes in Head and Neck Cancer Patients (OraRad). Oral Surg Oral Med Oral Pathol Oral Radiol. 2024 Mar;137(3):264–73.

Chapter 9
Radiation Dermatitis

Ana Carolina Prado Ribeiro, Karina Morais Faria, Thaís Bianca Brandão, Rafael Tomaz Gomes, and Gustavo Nader Marta

Disease Definition

Radiation dermatitis (RD) is one of the main adverse reactions resulting from exclusive or adjuvant radiotherapy (RT) in the head and neck region. It affects about 90–95% of patients in this context. The skin is a highly proliferating tissue that balances cell death and renewal. Continuous and subsequent exposure to ionizing radiation favors the development of an inflammatory reaction due to injury of the epidermal basal cells, endothelial cells, and vascular components, leading to the loss of skin self-renewal properties. Acute RD manifests as erythema, hyperpigmentation, and dry or moist desquamation.

RD typically manifests within 1–6 weeks of RT and may persist for 2–8 weeks following RT. During the initial week of treatment, with a daily fractionated dose of 2.0 Gy, patients typically do not experience significant discomfort. The clinical manifestation (Fig. 9.1) of skin erythema is observable 2–3 weeks following RT. Hyperpigmentation, desquamation, and a rash-like appearance may occur between 2 and 4 weeks after treatment has commenced. Patients may report that

A. C. P. Ribeiro · K. M. Faria
Dental Oncology Service, São Paulo State Cancer Institute, University of São Paulo Medical School, São Paulo, SP, Brazil

T. B. Brandão
Dental Oncology Service, São Paulo State Cancer Institute, University of São Paulo Medical School, São Paulo, SP, Brazil

Oral Medicine Department, Sírio-Libanês Hospital, São Paulo, SP, Brazil

R. T. Gomes (✉)
Department of Dermatology, Federal University of São Paulo, São Paulo, SP, Brazil

G. N. Marta
Radiotherapy Department, Sírio-Libanês Hospital, São Paulo, SP, Brazil

A. R. Santos-Silva et al. (eds.), *Photobiomodulation Therapy in Oral Medicine*, https://doi.org/10.1007/978-3-031-85048-6_9

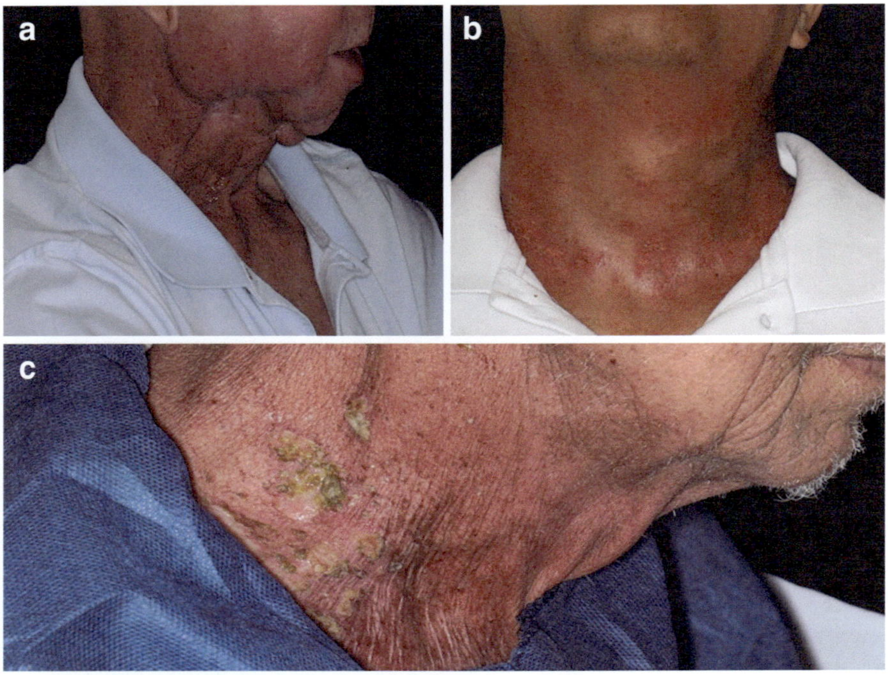

Fig. 9.1 (**a**) Facial and cervical skin erythema observed during second week of RT. (**b**) Cervical skin exhibits a red, warm, and rash-like appearance during the third week of RT. (**c**) Skin ulcers associate with exudate during RT

their skin feels sensitive, warm, and tight. Following the administration of cumulative RT doses reaching 30 Gy, patients may experience pain, pruritus, edema, ulcers, and exudate and crusting. These skin changes not only lead to significant discomfort and pain but also adversely impact the patient's quality of life. In severe cases, the symptomatic progression of RD can necessitate the temporary or permanent discontinuation of RT, thereby impacting therapeutic outcomes.

Diagnosis

- Clinical evaluation

Treatment

RD management should start with patient awareness regarding the skin care necessary to be performed before, after and during radiation treatment. This information will be instructed by radio-oncologists and nursing team (for those patients who will treat head and neck cancer (HNC) at hospital facilities). However, dentists who follow HNC patients for Oral mucositis (OM) prevention and treatment by using photobiomodulation therapy (PBMT) may endorse skin care guidance by instructing these individuals that topical drugs and any type of cosmetics must be removed before RT. In addition, dentists may advise patients to refrain from shaving the irradiated area until RD has healed. Besides, patients should be advised that the affected skin should not be scrubbed but gently washed. In summary, skin that is irradiated should be kept dry and clean for RT session.

Topical pharmacological (e.g., corticosteroids, triethanolamine cream, and silver-containing foam bandage) and non-pharmacological therapies (chamomile sugar-free iced tea) are used in the prevention and treatment of acute RD. Moisturizers can sooth the skin and attenuate irritation caused by RD.

A systematic review designed to evaluate the use of photobiomodulation (PBM) to prevent or treat RD in cancer patients undergoing RT, including only clinical trials, suggested a significant effect of PBM in preventing severe RD (Figs. 9.2 and 9.3). Table 9.1 displays the suggested PBM protocol for RD.

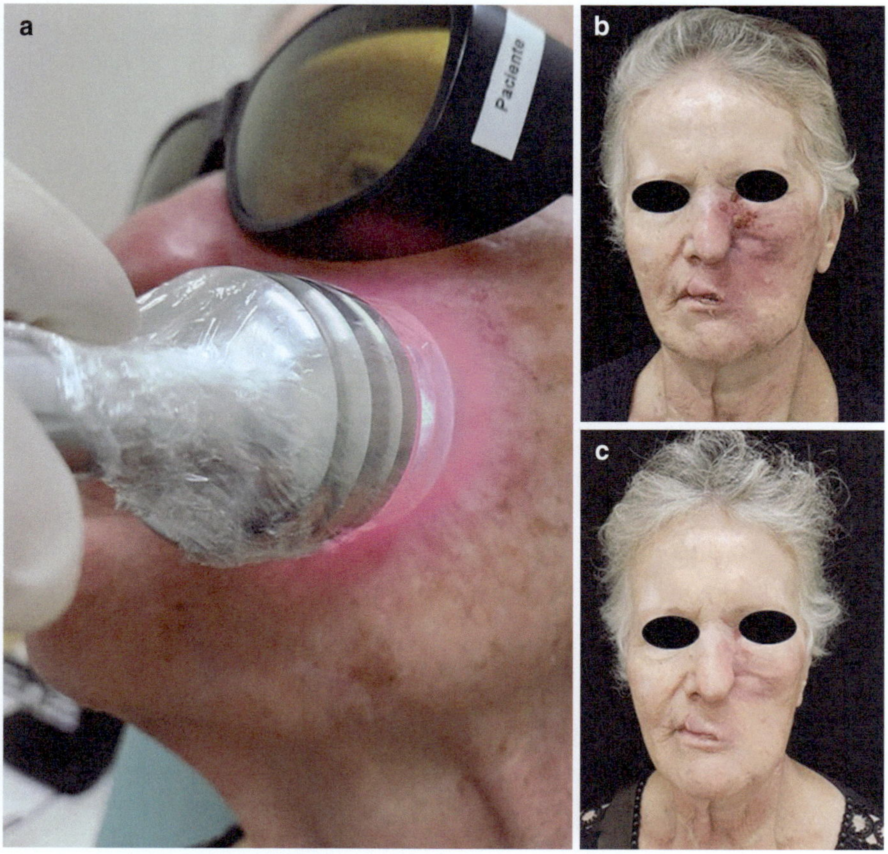

Fig. 9.2 (**a**) Extraoral PBMT with GEMINI ™. (Ultradent Products, Inc., South Jordan, UT, USA). (**b**) The initial clinical exam revealed facial skin exhibiting a red, warm, rash-like appearance, and ulcers. (**c**) RD healing after five sessions of extraoral PBMT

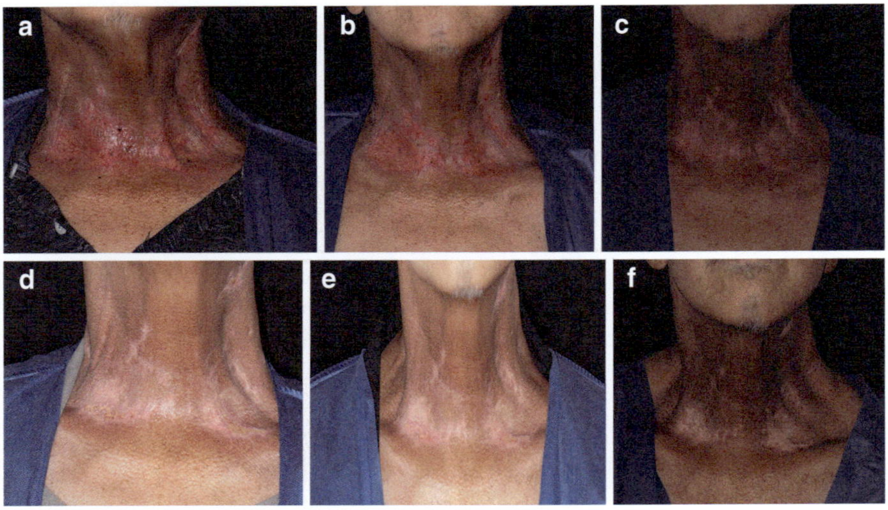

Fig. 9.3 (**a**). Severe RD. Initial clinical exam revealed cervical skin exhibiting edema, ulcers, exudate, and crusting. Extraoral PBMT, 1W, 5 points of application on cervical skin, 30 s/point (D1). (**b**) (D2). (**c**) (D3). (**d**) (D4). (**e**) (D5). (**f**) RD healing after five sessions of extraoral PBMT

Table 9.1 Photobiomodulation parameters suggested for treating radiation dermatitis

Wavelength (nm)		Red: 630–680	NIR: 810
Power (mW)		100	
Radiant energy (J)		3	
Fluence (J/cm^2)		Prevention: 2–3	Treatment: 4
Photonic fluence	(p.J/cm^2)	≈ 3.8–6.3	≈ 6
	(Einstein)	≈ 0.8–1.4	≈ 1.3
Exposure time (s/point)		30	
Spot location		Extraoral cutaneous surfaces on the radiation field where dermatitis is anticipated (often erythematous after RT)	
Treatment days		Prevention: start daily at the initiation of RT Treatment: continue treatment at least three times a week until recovery	

Treatment

- *Systemic Pharmacological Treatment*
  - Analgesics and anti-inflammatory drugs
  - It is recommended to discuss with the patient's radio-oncologist the prescription of analgesics and anti-inflammatory drugs to ensure the most suitable analgesic protocol. Physicians usually consider all steps of pain management scale when prescribing analgesics.
  - Pentoxifylline–tocopherol–clodronate combination (PENTOCLO)

- *Topical Pharmacological Treatment*
  - Moisturizers
  - Topical corticosteroids
  - Triethanolamine cream
  - Silver-containing foam bandage for ulcerative lesions (e.g., Mepilex®)
- *Miscellaneous*
  - Chamomile sugar-free iced tea
- *Photobiomodulation*

Funding This work was funded by São Paulo Research Foundation (FAPESP)—grant 16/22862-2.

Further Reading

Aguiar BRL, Guerra ENS, Normando AGC, Martins CC, Reis PEDD, Ferreira EB. Effectiveness of photobiomodulation therapy in radiation dermatitis: a systematic review and meta-analysis. Crit Rev Oncol Hematol. 2021 Jun;162:103349.

Bensadoun RJ. Photobiomodulation or low-level laser therapy in the management of cancer therapy-induced mucositis, dermatitis and lymphedema. Curr Opin Oncol. 2018 Jul;30(4):226–32.

Behroozian T, Bonomo P, Patel P, Kanee L, Finkelstein S, van den Hurk C, Chow E, Wolf JR, Multinational Association of Supportive Care in Cancer (MASCC) Oncodermatology Study Group Radiation Dermatitis Guidelines Working Group. Multinational Association of Supportive Care in Cancer (MASCC) clinical practice guidelines for the prevention and management of acute radiation dermatitis: international Delphi consensus-based recommendations. Lancet Oncol. 2023 Apr;24(4):e172–85.

Gobbo M, Rico V, Marta GN, Caini S, Ryan Wolf J, van den Hurk C, Beveridge M, Lam H, Bonomo P, Chow E, Behroozian T. Photobiomodulation therapy for the prevention of acute radiation dermatitis: a systematic review and meta-analysis. Support Care Cancer. 2023 Mar 23;31(4):227.

McQuestion M. Evidence-based skin care management in radiation therapy: clinical update. Semin Oncol Nurs. 2011 May;27(2):e1–17.

Robijns J, Lodewijckx J, Claes S, Van Bever L, Pannekoeke L, Censabella S, Bussé L, Colson D, Kaminski I, Broux V, Puts S, Vanmechelen S, Timmermans A, Noé L, Bulens P, Govers M, Maes A, Mebis J. Photobiomodulation therapy for the prevention of acute radiation dermatitis in head and neck cancer patients (DERMISHEAD trial). Radiother Oncol. 2021 May;158:268–75.

Tsai PC, Liu YC, Li TS, Hsu FT, Lee YH, Chiang IT, Chang Y, Lee CH. Clinical effect of moisturized skin care on radiation dermatitis of head and neck cancer. In Vivo. 2023 Nov–Dec;37(6):2776–85.

Wong RK, Bensadoun RJ, Boers-Doets CB, Bryce J, Chan A, Epstein JB, Eaby-Sandy B, Lacouture ME. Clinical practice guidelines for the prevention and treatment of acute and late radiation reactions from the MASCC Skin Toxicity Study Group. Support Care Cancer. 2013 Oct;21(10):2933–48.

Chapter 10
Medication-Related Osteonecrosis of Jaws

Luiz Alcino Monteiro Gueiros, Letícia Lang, Camila Barcellos Calderipe, Caique Mariano Pedroso, Thaís Cristina Esteves-Pereira, and Marcio Ajudarte Lopes

Disease Definition

Medication-related osteonecrosis of the jaw (MRONJ) is defined as necrotic bone tissue exposed or bone that can be probed through a fistula in the maxillofacial region that does not heal in ≈2 months manifested in a patient who has received antiresorptive therapy (e.g., bisphosphonates or denosumab) alone or in combination with immune modulators or antiangiogenic medications, with no history of radiation to the jaws or metastatic disease into the jaws. MRONJ may be associated with infection with or without intra- and extraoral fistula and bone fractures. Therefore, MRONJ may significantly impact to both the patient's quality of life and health care resources.

The pathogenesis of MRONJ is likely to be multifactorial and can involve a synergistic effect between local infection/trauma and decreased bone turnover after exposure to bone-modifying agents or antiangiogenic agents. Thus, the reasons that explain the specificity of the disease, which is almost exclusive to the jaws, are unclear, but hypotheses also include innate or acquired immunological dysfunction and genetic predisposition.

Therefore, dentists should be aware of patients receiving (1) antiresorptive or (2) antiangiogenic drugs because oral procedures that are related to surgical procedures

L. A. M. Gueiros (✉)
Clinical and Preventive Dentistry Department, Federal University of Pernambuco, Recife, PE, Brazil
e-mail: luiz.mgueiros@ufpe.br

L. Lang
Oncology and Radiotherapy Center of Londrina, Private Practice, Londrina, PR, Brazil

C. B. Calderipe · C. M. Pedroso · T. C. Esteves-Pereira · M. A. Lopes
Oral Diagnosis Department, Piracicaba Dental School, University of Campinas, Piracicaba, SP, Brazil

A. R. Santos-Silva et al. (eds.), *Photobiomodulation Therapy in Oral Medicine*,
https://doi.org/10.1007/978-3-031-85048-6_10

(e.g., tooth extraction and dental implant placement) or to odontogenic infections (such as endodontic and periodontal infections) may be associated with MRONJ. Not surprisingly, these procedures should be preferable performed before the initiation of those MRONJ-related medications. Moreover, dentists have an important impact in MRONJ prevention and diagnosis by practicing a minimal invasive philosophy and recognizing early signs of such undesired complication.

In this context, the American Society of Clinical Oncology and Cancer Care Ontario made the following recommendation: "A dental assessment is recommended, where feasible, before commencement of bisphosphonates, and any pending dental or oral health problems should be dealt with before starting treatment, if possible."

The stage of MRONJ is based on the clinical and radiographic findings (Table 10.1).

The incidence of MRONJ in patients receiving oral bisphosphonate is relatively low in literature, with a prevalence of up to 0.01%. However, ≈12% of MRONJ is reported for individuals receiving the intravenous drug and ≈16% in patients receiving a combination of bisphosphonates and antiangiogenics.

Antiresorptive Medications

Oral Bisphosphonates

The most common use of oral bisphosphonates is to treat osteoporosis and is frequently used to treat osteopenia and less common other conditions (such as Paget's disease of bone and osteogenesis imperfecta). Table 10.2 presents a selection of bisphosphonates used in medical practice to prevent bone loss. It is crucial to emphasize that dentists should conduct a comprehensive anamnesis prior to dental procedures, as patients are often unaware that oral bisphosphonates are linked to MRONJ. As these drugs are commonly used to treat osteoporosis and osteopenia, individuals may be aware that these drugs have an action like that of a calcium supplement.

Intravenous Bisphosphonates

Intravenous bisphosphonates are commonly used in oncology, mainly for hematological malignances (most frequently multiple myeloma), to control hypercalcemia of malignancy and to treat or prevent the progress of metastatic tumors to

Table 10.1 Staging classification of medication-related osteonecrosis of the jaw[a]

Stage	Definition
Risk Stage	No apparent necrotic bone in asymptomatic patients who have been treated with IV or oral antiresorptive or antiangiogenic therapy
Stage 0	Patients with no clinical evidence of necrotic bone, but present with nonspecific symptoms or clinical and radiographic findings
Stage 1	Exposed and necrotic bone, or fistulae that probe to bone, in patients who are asymptomatic and have no evidence of infection. These patients may also present with radiographic findings mentioned for Stage 0 which are localized to the alveolar bone region.
Stage 2	Exposed and necrotic bone, or fistulae that probe to bone, with evidence of infection. These patients are typically symptomatic. These patients may also present with radiographic findings mentioned for Stage 0 which are localized to the alveolar bone region.
Stage 3	Exposed and necrotic bone, or fistulae that probe to bone, with evidence of infection, and one or more of the following: exposed necrotic bone extending beyond the region of alveolar bone, i.e., inferior border and ramus in the mandible, maxillary sinus, and zygoma in the maxilla, pathologic fracture, extraoral fistula, oral antral/oral nasal communication, and osteolysis extending to the inferior border of the mandible or sinus floor

Symptoms: odontalgia not explained by an odontogenic cause; dull, aching bone pain in the body of the mandible, which may radiate to the temporomandibular joint region; sinus pain, which may be associated with inflammation and thickening of the maxillary sinus wall; altered neurosensory function
Clinical Findings: loosening of teeth not explained by chronic periodontal disease; periapical/periodontal fistula that is not associated with pulpal necrosis due to caries.
Radiographic Findings: alveolar bone loss or resorption not attributable to chronic periodontal disease changes to trabecular pattern—dense woven bone and persistence of unremodeled bone in extraction sockets; regions of osteosclerosis involving the alveolar bone and/or the surrounding basilar bone; thickening/obscuring of periodontal ligament (thickening of the lamina dura and decreased size of the periodontal ligament space)

[a]Table extracted from Ruggiero SL, Dodson TB, Aghaloo T, Carlson ER, Ward BB, Kademani D. American Association of Oral and Maxillofacial Surgeons' Position Paper on Medication-Related Osteonecrosis of the Jaws-2022 Update. J Oral Maxillofac Surg. 2022 May;80(5):920–943

bone tissue. These medications provide several clinical benefits, including the prevention to pathologic fractures and spinal cord compression—which significantly reduces patients' mobility—and reduce need for radiation or surgery to bone. Table 10.2 also displays some intravenous bisphosphonates used in oncology.

It is important to consider that, although at a lower dose and frequency, intravenous bisphosphonates are also increasingly being recommended to treat osteoporosis, having been an option for patients with low adherence or response to oral medications.

Table 10.2 Commercially available antiresorptive drugs[a]

Antiresorptive	Category	Brand names	Administration
Etidronate	Non-nitrogen bisphosphonate	Didronel®	Oral
Tiludronate	Non-nitrogen bisphosphonate	Skelid®	Oral
Clodronate	Non-nitrogen bisphosphonate	Clasteon®, Bonefos®, Osphos®	Oral/IV
Alendronate	Nitrogen bisphosphonate	Fosamax®	Oral
Ibandronate	Nitrogen bisphosphonate	Bandrone®, Boniva®	Oral/IV
Residronate	Nitrogen bisphosphonate	Actonel®	Oral
Pamidronate	Nitrogen bisphosphonate	Aredia®	IV
Zoledronate	Nitrogen bisphosphonate	Zometa®, Aclasta®	IV
Denosumab	RANKL inhibitor	Prolia®, Xgeva®	Subcutaneous

IV: intravenous

[a]Table adapted from Diagnóstico e tratamento odontológico para pacientes oncológicos. Editors: Thaís Bianca Brandão, Cesar Augusto Migliorati, Alan Roger Santos-Silva et al.; 2021; GEN Guanabara Koogan; p. 192; ISBN: 978-8-595-15121-5

RANK Ligand Inhibitor (Denosumab)

It is an antiresorptive agent that exists as a fully humanized antibody against RANK ligand (RANK-L) and inhibits osteoclast function and associated bone resorption. The most common drug from this class of medications is denosumab (e.g., Prolia® and Xgeva®).

Dentists should be aware when evaluating an osteoporotic patient because denosumab may be commonly administered subcutaneously, every 6 months, to reduce their risk to vertebral, non-vertebral, and hip fractures. Denosumab is also effective to manage metastatic bone disease from solid tumors when administered monthly. Wyost© and Jubbonti© are biosimilars to denosumab that can be interchangeably used with denosumab, and the same risk profile should be expected.

Interestingly, in contrast to bisphosphonates, RANK ligand inhibitors do not bind to bone, and their effects on bone remodeling are mostly diminished within 6 months of treatment interruption or break. Despite this, denosumab has an increased osteolysis inhibitory action, which makes the prevalence of MRONJ among its users at least as high as among bisphosphonate users.

Antiangiogenic Medications

Angiogenesis inhibitors interfere with the formation of new blood vessels by binding to various signaling molecules disrupting the angiogenesis signaling cascade. These novel medications have demonstrated efficacy in the treatment of gastrointestinal tumors, renal cell carcinomas, neuroendocrine tumors, and others.

Diagnosis

- Clinical and imaging evaluation
- Medical and dental history

Treatment

Treatment must be individualized and depends on the patient's systemic conditions and the staging of the disease. In early cases, the treatment is usually more conservative (oral antibacterial mouth rinse, antibiotic therapy, and pain control). In cases of more advanced disease, treatment is always very challenging and often requires surgical intervention. The combination of therapies has shown good success rates in the management of MRONJ, and photobiomodulation (PBM) has been an important tool in both initial and advanced stages.

Anecdotal evidence has suggested PBM as an adjuvant treatment in cases of MRONJ. PBM has been demonstrated to provide a significant improvement in the signs of inflammation, pain, and bone/soft tissue repair. It is a noninvasive therapy that stimulates angiogenesis, enhancing oxygen supply to the affected tissues. This may improve bone remodeling, which is compromised by antiresorptive drugs. PBM also plays an important role in the management of side effects resulting from MRONJ, such as paresthesia and trismus. Avoid using PBM as single therapy. Combined use, as suggested, may improve clinical results.

It is crucial to highlight that an accurate diagnosis is a fundamental prerequisite for the effective management of MRONJ. It is important to note that bone metastases and certain odontogenic conditions may present with similar symptoms or clinical manifestations, which may preclude the use of PBM.

Therefore, it is important to observe if PBM applications are promoting positive results in MRONJ treatment. If MRONJ area is increasing, the surgical debridement is encouraged, and PBM may be associated to enhance the postoperatory recovery. Table 10.3 displays the suggested PBM parameters for MRONJ.

Table 10.3 Photobiomodulation parameters suggested for treating medication-related osteonecrosis of the jaw

Wavelength (nm)		Red: 660	NIR: 780–810
Power (mW)		100	
Radiant energy (J)		3/point	
Fluence (J/cm^2)		3	
Photonic fluence	(p.J/cm^2)	≈ 5.7	≈ 4.5–4.8
	(Einstein)	≈ 1.2	≈ 1
Exposure time (s/point)		30	
Spot location		Right below the bone margin (at vestibular and lingual/palatine), in contact, at a 90-degree angle with the tissue, with equidistant points 1 cm apart	
Treatment days		Three sessions/week[a]	

[a]Selected studies describe PBM regimes from 10 to 12 sessions. Patient's symptoms may demand modifications to this strategy. Therefore, consider repeating until positive response since there is no scientific evidence contraindicating PBM continuity. However, surgical debridement is encouraged if MRONJ area is increasing. PBM may be associated to enhance the postoperatory recovery

Treatment

- *Systemic Pharmacological Treatment*
  - Opioid analgesics
  - It is recommended to discuss with the patient's oncologist or palliative doctor the prescription of opioids to ensure the most suitable analgesic protocol. Physicians usually consider all steps of pain management scale when prescribing analgesics.
  - Antibiotic therapy
  - Amoxicillin/clavulanic acid or clindamycin for 7–14 days is a suggestion to resolve infections. Infections are important to treat not only to avoid urgent conditions but also to improve results of surgical debridement
- *Topical Pharmacological Treatment*
  - Oral antibacterial mouthwashes
  - Chlorhexidine 0.12%, for 1 min, every 12 h. Clinicians should maintain mouthwash use until infection is controlled.
- *Surgical Treatment*
  - Cautious debridement or sequestrectomies of exposed necrotic bone
- *Antimicrobial photodynamic therapy* (see the specific chapter for more info)
- *Photobiomodulation*

Further Reading

Almeida MVDC, Moura AC, Santos L, Gominho L, Cavalcanti UDNT, Romeiro K. Photodynamic therapy as an adjunct in the treatment of medication-related osteonecrosis of the jaw: a case report. J Lasers Med Sci. 2021 Mar 8;12:e12.

El Mobadder M, Grzech-Lesniak Z, El Mobadder W, Rifai M, Ghandour M, Nammour S. Management of medication-related osteonecrosis of the jaw with photobiomodulation and minimal surgical intervention. Dent J (Basel). 2023;11(5):127.

Razavi P, Jafari A, Vescovi P, Fekrazad R. Efficacy of adjunctive photobiomodulation in the management of medication-related osteonecrosis of the jaw: a systematic review. Photobiomodul Photomed Laser Surg. 2022 Dec;40(12):777–91.

Tartaroti NC, Marques MM, Naclério-Homem MDG, Migliorati CA, Zindel Deboni MC. Antimicrobial photodynamic and photobiomodulation adjuvant therapies for prevention and treatment of medication-related osteonecrosis of the jaws: case series and long-term follow-up. Photodiagnosis Photodyn Ther. 2020;29:101651.

Tenore G, Zimbalatti A, Rocchetti F, Graniero F, Gaglioti D, Mohsen A, Caputo M, Lollobrigida M, Lamazza L, De Biase A, Barbato E, Romeo U. Management of medication-related osteonecrosis of the jaw (MRONJ) using leukocyte- and platelet-rich fibrin (L-PRF) and photobiomodulation: a retrospective study. J Clin Med. 2020;9:3505.

Torres AA, de Freitas BL, Carneiro PP, de Sousa ALA, Arêa Leão Ferraz MÂ, de Pinho Mendes J, Costa ALF, Pinto ASB. Medication-related osteonecrosis of the jaw and low-level laser therapy as adjuvant treatment: a case report. J Lasers Med Sci. 2020 Fall;11(4):497–9.

Chapter 11
Osteoradionecrosis

Luiz Alcino Monteiro Gueiros, Letícia Lang, Rogério de Andrade Elias, Maria Cecília Querido de Oliveira, and Aljomar José Vechiato Filho

Disease Definition

Treatments of head and neck cancer include surgery, radiotherapy (RT), chemotherapy (CT), or the combination of these methods. RT is frequently performed after operable oral tumors (classified as adjuvant) or exclusively for non-operable lesions (tumor infiltration of carotid artery, for example) and patients who refuse surgery (classified as exclusive) or in combination with CT for oro-, naso-, and hypopharyngeal tumors (classified as concomitant).

Despite its very effective performance in directly and indirectly destroying tumor cells, it results in acute and chronic side effects (also named as toxicities), in oral tissues. Unfortunately, irradiation decreases the capacity of bone tissue repair in maxilla and mandible, which may result in one of the most relevant late toxicities related to RT of head and neck region: the osteoradionecrosis (ORN) of the jaw.

ORN is defined as exposed necrotic bone tissue that fails to heal over a period of 3 months without evidence of persisting or recurrent tumor. Clinical signs and

L. A. M. Gueiros
Clinical and Preventive Dentistry Department, Federal University of Pernambuco, Recife, PE, Brazil

L. Lang
Oncology and Radiotherapy Center of Londrina, Private Practice, Londrina, PR, Brazil

R. de Andrade Elias
Oral Diagnosis Department, Piracicaba Dental School, University of Campinas, Piracicaba, SP, Brazil

M. C. Q. de Oliveira · A. J. Vechiato Filho (✉)
Dental Oncology Service, Instituto do Cancer do Estado de Sao Paulo (ICESP), University of São Paulo, São Paulo, SP, Brazil
e-mail: aljomar.filho@hc.fm.usp.br

A. R. Santos-Silva et al. (eds.), *Photobiomodulation Therapy in Oral Medicine*,
https://doi.org/10.1007/978-3-031-85048-6_11

Table 11.1 Staging system for osteoradionecrosis of the mandible[a]

Stage	Definition
Stage 0	Exposure of mandibular bone for less than 1 month; no distinct changes on plain radiographs (panoramic radiograph or periapical film)
Stage 1	Exposure of mandibular bone for at least 1–3 months; no distinct changes on plain radiographs (panoramic radiograph or periapical film). Asymptomatic otherwise, e.g., no pain or presence of cutaneous fistulas (I A), or symptomatic, e.g., pain or presence of cutaneous fistulas (I B)
Stage 2	Exposure of mandibular bone for at least one month; distinct changes present on plain radiographs (panoramic radiograph or periapical film), but not involving the lower border of the mandible. Asymptomatic otherwise, e.g., no pain or presence of cutaneous fistulas (II A), or symptomatic, e.g., pain or presence of cutaneous fistulas (II B)
Stage 3	Exposure of mandibular bone for at least 1 month; distinct changes on plain radiographs (panoramic radiograph or periapical film), involving the lower border of the mandible, irrespective of any other signs and symptoms

Note: In case of doubt about the presence and/or extent of radiographical bone involvement, the lower stage should be allotted

[a]Table adapted from Karagozoglu KH, Dekker HA, Rietveld D, de Bree R, Schulten EA, Kantola S, Forouzanfar T, van der Waal I. Proposal for a new staging system for osteoradionecrosis of the mandible. Med Oral Patol Oral Cir Bucal. 2014 Sep 1;19(5):e433–7

symptoms of ORN may include ulceration or necrosis of the mucosa with bone exposure, pain, trismus, and infection with or without suppuration.

Many risk factors are related to higher chances to developed ORN after the treatment, such as radiotherapy with curative purpose, which will deliver high doses of radiation (≈70 Gy), presence of dental caries, periodontal disease, poorly adapted prosthesis, oral surgery (such as dental extractions and implant placement after RT), smoking and drinking habits during and after RT, and nutritional status. Despite the well-known risk factors and careful dental practice, ORN may also occur spontaneously.

Some lines of evidence support that a comprehensive evaluation by an experienced dental clinician for all patients undergoing head and neck RT is imperative to establish a dental treatment plan focused on resolving odontogenic sources of infection. This strategy is suggested to reduce the risk of ORN and other radiation-related adverse effects on the oral cavity, as well.

The stages of ORN are divided according to the clinical and radiographic features of the condition (see Table 11.1). The treatment proposed for each patient will depend on several factors such as the stage of the ORN, the oncological status of the patient, and the availability of treatment available in medical centers, among others.

Diagnosis

- Clinical and imaging evaluation
- Medical and dental history

Treatment

Treatments to ORN include nonsurgical debridement, antibiotic therapy, hyperbaric oxygenation, pentoxifylline–tocopherol–clodronate combination (PENTOCLO), and surgery. Photobiomodulation therapy (PBMT) associated with antimicrobial photodynamic therapy (aPDT) has also been reported as alternative strategies that can be added to the management flowchart.

The analgesic effect of photobiomodulation (PBM) may be useful for patients with ORN although this complication is normally a non-painful condition per say. However, ORN can be associated with pain if its severity leads to a bone fracture of the mandible (Fig. 11.1), infection of the necrotic bone with suppuration or fistulas, or even when the necrotic bone is traumatizing the tongue (Fig. 11.2), for example.

The analgesic effect is created by the inhibition of the electrophysiological activity of the irradiated nerve, increasing the release of neurotransmitter that is associated with pain relief. Therefore, patient's quality of life may be maintained as good as possible through pain control, while clinician's efforts are focused on wound healing. Furthermore, patients with controlled pain will be more likely to preserve basic oral functions, such as eating, drinking, swallowing, and talking.

The effectiveness of PBM is supported by studies that evaluated its effects on the healing process of the oral mucosa by inducing the proliferation and transformation of fibroblasts and myofibroblasts. PBM also increases the blood flow by angiogenesis through revascularization and capillary growth, which enhances nutrient and oxygen supply to the affected tissues, potentially improving osteogenesis and bone

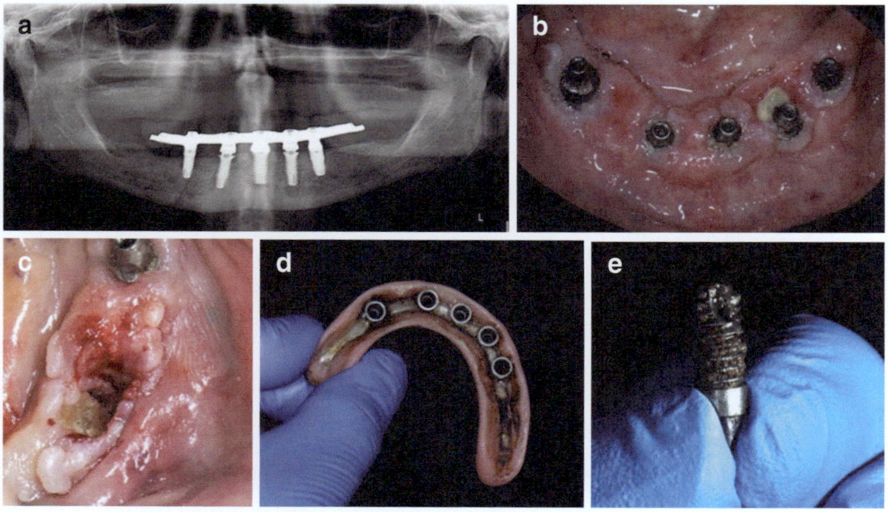

Fig. 11.1 Stage 1B ORN associated with dental implants. (**a**) Panoramic radiograph with no distinct changes. (**b**) Exposed mandibular bone. (**c**) Exposed mandibular bone after implant removal. (**d**) Implant-supported prosthesis removed due to infection and necrosis of mandibular bone. (**e**) Necrotic bone in the removed dental implant

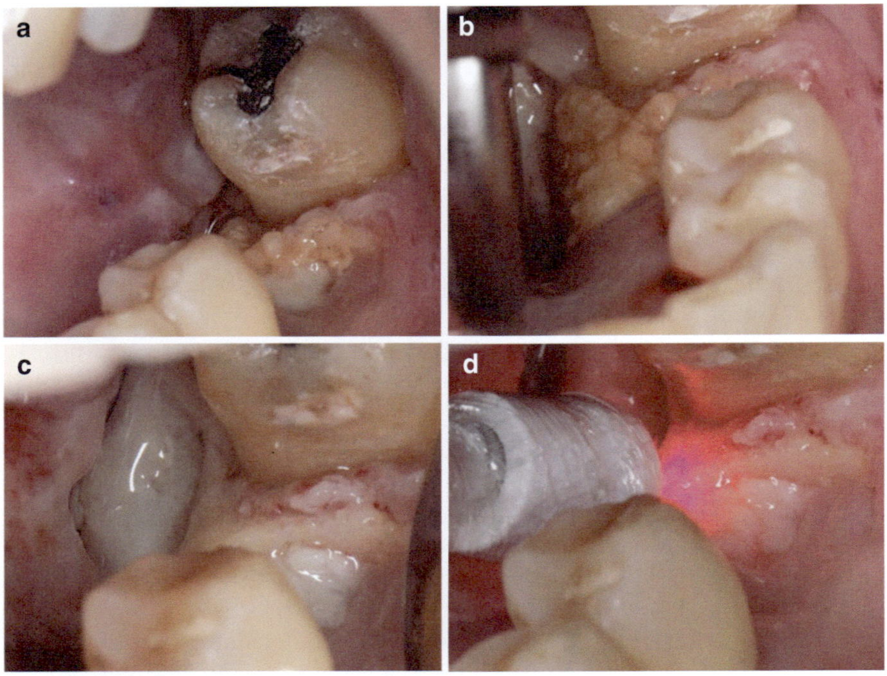

Fig. 11.2 Exposed necrotic bone traumatizing the tongue. (**a**) Exposed necrotic bone in the right posterior mandible. (**b**, **c**) Painful ulcer in the lateral tongue due to necrotic bone trauma. (**d**) Photobiomodulation using red laser (660 nm) to exposed necrotic mandibular bone

remodeling. PBM may also be indicated for the management of side effects resulting from ORN, such as paresthesia and trismus. Besides, PBMT is noninvasive, and the absence of significant adverse effects highlights its safety and promising potential to be incorporated into therapy strategies for ORN management (Table 11.2). Currently, MASCC/ASCO does not support PBM to prevent ORN for patients undergoing dental procedures after head and neck RT due to limited evidence available. It should be considered in a case-by-case definition. PBM can be of relevance in advanced painful cases under exclusive palliation, where surgical interventions are not considered.

Table 11.2 Photobiomodulation parameters suggested for treating osteoradionecrosis

Wavelength (nm)		Red: 660	NIR: 810
Power (mW)		100	
Radiant energy (J)		1/point	3/point
Fluence (J/cm^2)		1	3
Photonic fluence	(p.J/cm^2)	≈ 1.9	≈ 4.5
	(Einstein)	≈ 0.4	≈ 1
Exposure time (s/point)		10	30
Spot location		Right below the bone margin (at vestibular and lingual/palatine), in contact, at a 90-degree angle with the tissue, with equidistant points 1 cm apart	
Treatment days		Three sessions/week[a]	

[a]There is no recommendation for treatment duration. Patient's symptoms may demand modifications to this strategy. Therefore, consider repeating until positive response since there is no scientific evidence contraindicating PBM continuity. However, surgical debridement is encouraged if ORN area is increasing. PBM with red laser may be associated to enhance the postoperatory recovery

Treatment

- *Systemic Pharmacological Treatment*
  - Analgesics
    It is recommended to discuss with the patient's head and neck surgeon, radio-oncologist, oncologist, or palliative doctor the prescription of opioids to ensure the most suitable analgesic protocol. Physicians usually consider all steps of pain management scale when prescribing analgesics.
  - Antibiotic therapy
    Amoxicillin/clavulanic acid or clindamycin for 7–14 days is a suggestion to resolve infections. Infections are important to treat not only to avoid urgent conditions but also to improve results of surgical debridement.
  - Pentoxifylline-tocopherol-clodronate combination
- *Topical Pharmacological Treatment*
  - Oral antibacterial mouthwashes
  - Chlorhexidine 0.12%, for 1 min, every 12 h. Clinicians should maintain mouthwash use until infection is controlled.
- *Surgical treatment*
  - Cautious debridement or sequestrectomies of exposed necrotic bone
  - Extensive surgical resections with or without reconstruction performed by head and neck surgeons

- *Miscellaneous*
  - Hyperbaric oxygenation
- *Photobiomodulation*
- *Antimicrobial photodynamic therapy* (see the specific chapter for more info)

Further Reading

Chronopoulos A, Zarra T, Ehrenfeld M, Otto S. Osteoradionecrosis of the jaws: definition, epidemiology, staging and clinical and radiological findings. A concise review. Int Dent J. 2018;68:22–30.

da Silva TMV, Melo TS, de Alencar RC, Pereira JRD, Leão JC, Silva IHM, Gueiros LA. Photobiomodulation for mucosal repair in patients submitted to dental extraction after head and neck radiation therapy: a double-blind randomized pilot study. Support Care Cancer. 2021 Mar;29(3):1347–54.

Magalhães IA, Forte CPF, Viana TSA, Teófilo CR, Lima Verde RMB, Magalhães DP, Praxedes Neto RAL, Lima RA, Dantas TS. Photobiomodulation and antimicrobial photodynamic therapy as adjunct in the treatment and prevention of osteoradionecrosis of the jaws: a case report. Photodiagnosis Photodyn Ther. 2020;31:101959.

Peterson DE, Koyfman SA, Yarom N, Lynggaard CD, Ismaila N, Forner LE, Fuller CD, Mowery YM, Murphy BA, Watson E, Yang DH, Alajbeg I, Bossi P, Fritz M, Futran ND, Gelblum DY, King E, Ruggiero S, Smith DK, Villa A, Wu JS, Saunders D. Prevention and management of osteoradionecrosis in patients with head and neck cancer treated with radiation therapy: ISOO-MASCC-ASCO guideline. J Clin Oncol. 2024 May 1:JCO2302750.

Ribeiro GH, Minamisako MC, Rath IBDS, Santos AMB, Simões A, Pereira KCR, Grando LJ. Osteoradionecrosis of the jaws: case series treated with adjuvant low-level laser therapy and antimicrobial photodynamic therapy. J Appl Oral Sci. 2018;26:e20170172.

Chapter 12
Hyposalivation Induced by Radiotherapy

Luiz Alcino Monteiro Gueiros, Ana Carolina Prado Ribeiro, Marcio Ajudarte Lopes, and Regina Maria Holanda de Mendonça

Disease Definition

Hyposalivation induced by radiotherapy (RT) is high prevalent adverse reaction of head and neck RT. The glandular tissues are damaged by irradiation, resulting in reduced salivary flow and xerostomia complaints. Xerostomia affects about 80–93% of patients undergoing head and neck RT, starting as an acute and maintaining as a long-lasting adverse event. The loss of gland function is progressive during the RT treatment course and is associated with higher doses of radiation. However, in pediatric and adolescent patients, a reduction in salivary flow rate at lower doses of radiation has been observed. Permanent damage to glandular tissues may occur due to RT.

Diagnosis

- Clinical evaluation
- Radiation history
- Salivary flow rate evaluation (sialometry) (Table 12.1)

L. A. M. Gueiros
Clinical and Preventive Dentistry Department, Federal University of Pernambuco, Recife, PE, Brazil

A. C. P. Ribeiro
Dental Oncology Service, São Paulo State Cancer Institute, University of São Paulo Medical School, São Paulo, SP, Brazil

M. A. Lopes
Oral Diagnosis Department, Piracicaba Dental School, University of Campinas, Piracicaba, SP, Brazil

R. M. Holanda de Mendonça (✉)
Dentistry Department, Boldrini Children's Hospital, Campinas, SP, Brazil

A. R. Santos-Silva et al. (eds.), *Photobiomodulation Therapy in Oral Medicine*, https://doi.org/10.1007/978-3-031-85048-6_12

Table 12.1 References value for sialometry[a]

	Normal salivary flow rate	Hyposalivation
Stimulated	1.5–2.0 mL/min	≤ 0.5–0.7 mL/min
Non-stimulated	0.3–0.4 mL/min	≤ 0.1 mL/min

[a]Table adapted from Clinical Decision Making in Oral Medicine: a concise guide to diagnosis and treatment. Editors: Alan Roger Santos-Silva, Márcio Ajudarte Lopes, João Figueira Scarini et al.; 2023; Springer Cham; p. 216; ISBN: 978-3-031-14945-0

Table 12.2 Photobiomodulation parameters suggested for treating hyposalivation induced by radiotherapy

Wavelength (nm)		Red: 660	NIR: 810
Power (mW)		100	
Radiant energy (J)		3/point	
Fluence (J/cm²)		3	
Photonic fluence	(p.J/cm²)	≈ 1.9	≈ 1.5
	(Einstein)	≈ 0.4	≈ 0.3
Exposure time (s/point)		30	
Spot location		Intraoral: two points on each sublingual gland. Minor salivary glands may be irradiated Extraoral: six points on each parotid gland and three points on each submandibular gland	
Treatment days		Every day or alternate days from the first day of RT until end of treatment	

Treatment

Management of RT-induced hyposalivation can initiate with the prevention of salivary gland damage using pharmacological radioprotectors, such as amifostine and cell growth factors. Sialagogues, particularly bethanechol, have shown efficacy in preserving residual salivary gland function when used during the radiation treatment. Also, acupuncture has been reported as an alternative intervention during the radiation therapy, being able to reduce RT-induced salivary gland dysfunction.

The interventions to manage the established hyposalivation are often less effective. Pilocarpine is suggested to slightly improve the salivary gland function, with minor impact on the symptom relief. The same applies to acupuncture. Saliva substitutes based on carboxymethylcellulose, mucin, or xanthan gum can be prescribed for symptomatic relief when used topically. Various substances can be used to stimulate saliva production, including gustatory stimulant tablets or chewing gums, as well as vegetables and fruits for mechanical stimulation.

During RT treatment, photobiomodulation has been used as a preventive approach to increase unstimulated salivary flow in head and neck irradiated patients affected by hyposalivation (Table 12.2 and Fig. 12.1).

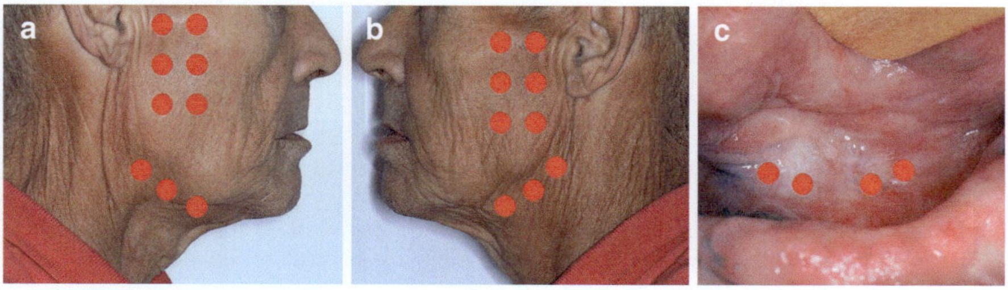

Fig. 12.1 Spot location for laser irradiation. (**a**, **b**) Six points on each parotid gland and three points on each submandibular gland. (**c**) Two points on each sublingual gland (note: this patient has undergone surgical resection of a squamous cell carcinoma on the tongue)

Treatment

- *Systemic Pharmacological Treatment*
  - Amifostine
  - Cell growth factors
  - Pilocarpine
  - Bethanechol (parasympathomimetic drugs)
- *Topical Pharmacological Treatment*
  - Pilocarpine
  - Saliva substitutes
- *Miscellaneous*
  - Mechanical/gustatory stimulants
  - Acupuncture
- *Photobiomodulation*

Funding This work was funded by São Paulo Research Foundation (FAPESP)—grants 16/22862-2 and 18/04657-8.

Further Reading

Heiskanen V, Zadik Y, Elad S. Photobiomodulation therapy for cancer treatment-related salivary gland dysfunction: a systematic review. Photobiomodul Photomed Laser Surg. 2020 Jun;38(6):340–7.

Hong C, Jensen SB, Vissink A, Bonomo P, Santos-Silva AR, Gueiros LA, Epstein JB, Elad S. MASCC/ISOO Clinical practice statement: management of salivary gland hypofunction and xerostomia in cancer patients. Support Care Cancer. 2024 Jul 25;32(8):548. Erratum in: Support Care Cancer. 2024 Nov 9;32(12):779.

Louzeiro GC, Cherubini K, de Figueiredo MAZ, Salum FG. Effect of photobiomodulation on salivary flow and composition, xerostomia and quality of life of patients during head and neck radiotherapy in short term follow-up: a randomized controlled clinical trial. J Photochem Photobiol B. 2020 Aug;209:111933.

Louzeiro GC, Teixeira DDS, Cherubini K, de Figueiredo MAZ, Salum FG. Does laser photobiomodulation prevent hyposalivation in patients undergoing head and neck radiotherapy? A systematic review and meta-analysis of controlled trials. Crit Rev Oncol Hematol. 2020 Dec;156:103115.

Marangoni-Lopes L, Rodrigues LP, Mendonça RH, Nobre-Dos Santos M. Radiotherapy changes salivary properties and impacts quality of life of children with Hodgkin disease. Arch Oral Biol. 2016 Dec;72:99–105.

Mercadante V, Al Hamad A, Lodi G, Porter S, Fedele S. Interventions for the management of radiotherapy-induced xerostomia and hyposalivation: a systematic review and meta-analysis. Oral Oncol. 2017 Mar;66:64–74.

Mercadante V, Jensen SB, Smith DK, Bohlke K, Bauman J, Brennan MT, Coppes RP, Jessen N, Malhotra NK, Murphy B, Rosenthal DI, Vissink A, Wu J, Saunders DP, Peterson DE. Salivary gland hypofunction and/or xerostomia induced by nonsurgical cancer therapies: ISOO/MASCC/ASCO Guideline. J Clin Oncol. 2021 Sep 1;39(25):2825–43.

Palma LF, Gonnelli FAS, Marcucci M, Dias RS, Giordani AJ, Segreto RA, Segreto HRC. Impact of low-level laser therapy on hyposalivation, salivary pH, and quality of life in head and neck cancer patients post-radiotherapy. Lasers Med Sci. 2017 May;32(4):827–32.

Schulz RE, Bonzanini LIL, Ortigara GB, Soldera EB, Danesi CC, Antoniazzi RP, Ferrazzo KL. Prevalence of hyposalivation and associated factors in survivors of head and neck cancer treated with radiotherapy. J Appl Oral Sci. 2021 Apr 19;29:e20200854.

Vissink A, Mitchell JB, Baum BJ, Limesand KH, Jensen SB, Fox PC, Elting LS, Langendijk JA, Coppes RP, Reyland ME. Clinical management of salivary gland hypofunction and xerostomia in head-and-neck cancer patients: successes and barriers. Int J Radiat Oncol Biol Phys. 2010 Nov 15;78(4):983–91.

Chapter 13
Hyposalivation Induced by Graft Versus Host Disease

Aljomar José Vechiato Filho, Ana Carolina Prado Ribeiro, Maria Cecília Querido de Oliveira, Vinícius Rabelo Torregrossa, Thaís Bianca Brandão, and Joel B. Epstein

Disease Definition

Graft-versus-Host Disease (GvHD) is a common and severe complication that can occur following allogenic HSCT (alloHSCT) for the treatment of a variety of malignant and nonmalignant hematologic conditions and some solid tumors. It can affect one or more systems. The disease has two forms, acute (aGvHD) and chronic (cGvHD), primarily distinguished by clinical features. The oral cavity is commonly affected by cGvHD, with a prevalence of 45–83%, resulting in oral mucositis with a lichenoid pattern, immune-mediated salivary gland dysfunction and orofacial sclerosis. Hyposalivation is a recognized complication of alloHSCT. In this population, salivary dysfunction can be found because of initial damage caused by the conditioning regimens toxicity, alone or in combination with total body irradiation, and to the presence of oral cGvHD. Decreased salivary flow increases the risk of opportunistic infections, caries, dysphagia, dysgeusia, and other oral complications.

A. J. Vechiato Filho · A. C. P. Ribeiro · M. C. Q. de Oliveira
Dental Oncology Service, São Paulo State Cancer Institute, University of São Paulo Medical School, São Paulo, SP, Brazil

V. R. Torregrossa (✉)
UniFTC University Center, Salvador, BA, Brazil

T. B. Brandão
Dental Oncology Service, São Paulo State Cancer Institute, University of São Paulo Medical School, São Paulo, SP, Brazil

Oral Medicine Department, Sírio-Libanês Hospital, São Paulo, SP, Brazil

J. B. Epstein
Cedars-Sinai Health System, Los Angeles, CA, USA

City of Hope National Medical Center, Duarte, CA, USA

A. R. Santos-Silva et al. (eds.), *Photobiomodulation Therapy in Oral Medicine*,
https://doi.org/10.1007/978-3-031-85048-6_13

Table 13.1 Photobiomodulation parameters suggested for treating hyposalivation induced by cGVHD

Wavelength (nm)		Red: 660	NIR: 810
Power (mW)		100	
Radiant energy (J)		3/point	
Fluence (J/cm^2)		3	
Photonic fluence	($p.J/cm^2$)	≈ 5.7	≈ 4.5
	(Einstein)	≈ 1.2	≈ 1.0
Exposure time (s/point)		30	
Spot location		Intraoral: two points on each sublingual gland. Minor salivary glands may be irradiated Extraoral: six points on each parotid gland and three points on each submandibular gland	
Treatment days		Initially, twice weekly sessions for 4 weeks and then gradually reducing the frequency of treatment until significant or total resolution of symptoms	

Diagnosis

- Clinical and histological evaluation
- GvHD diagnosis
- Salivary flow rate evaluation (sialometry) (see Table 13.1 from the Hyposalivation Induced by Radiotherapy chapter)
- Minor salivary gland biopsy

Treatment

Management of oral cGvHD should be considered in the overall management of GvHD, which may require systemic immunomodulatory medications. Systemic therapy might suppress dry mouth associated with oral cGvHD. However, topical therapies are the most effective strategy to treat oral cGVHD symptoms, and it could be combined with systemic therapy for greater results. In patients with persistent oral symptoms, pharmacological and non-pharmacological approaches may be beneficial for management of dry mouth.

For hyposalivation induced by oral cGvHD, first measures include encourage patients to increase water intake during the day and mealtime. Chewing gum can provide masticatory stimulation to glands, resulting in a momentary increase in salivary flow. Saliva substitutes can be used to temporarily reduce xerostomia, but they must be reapplied frequently to provide satisfactory results. If all the non-pharmacological measures implemented above have no effect, systemic administration of pilocarpine and cevimeline can be prescribed and have shown positive results, but data in cGvHD population is scarce.

Photobiomodulation (PBM) is a non-pharmacological, safe, and comfortable treatment that has not only been shown to increase the salivary flow in cGvHD patients (Table 13.1) but also has had positive results in controlling mucosal cGvHD and reducing orofacial tissue fibrosis. However, due to the increased risk for oral cancer in alloHSCT patients, a frequent oral examination also focused on oral cancer screening is recommended. Therefore, PBM can be used carefully to treat oral cGvHD considering that there is an adequate indication and accurate diagnosis of mucosal changes commonly found in alloHSCT patients.

Treatment

- *Systemic Pharmacological Treatment for hyposalivation induced by cGVHD*
  - Pilocarpine
  - Cevimeline
- *Topical Pharmacological Treatment for hyposalivation induced by cGVHD*
  - Saliva substitutes (lozenges, patches, rinses, and gels)
- *Miscellaneous*
  - Increase water intake
  - Mechanical/gustatory stimulants (e.g., chewing gum and sugar-free candy)
- *Photobiomodulation*

Further Reading

Epstein JB, Raber-Durlacher JE, Epstein GL, Hazenberg MD, Tzachanis D, Spielberger RT. Chronic oral graft-versus-host disease: induction and maintenance therapy with photobiomodulation therapy. Support Care Cancer. 2021 Mar;29(3):1387–94.

Epstein JB, Raber-Durlacher JE, Lill M, Linhares YP, Chang J, Barasch A, Slief RI, Geuke M, Zecha JA, Milstein DM, Tzachanis D. Photobiomodulation therapy in the management of chronic oral graft-versus-host disease. Support Care Cancer. 2017 Feb;25(2):357–64.

Gervazio TC, Silva JK, Evangelista K, Cavalcanti MGP, Silva MAGS, Yamamoto-Silva FP, Silva BSF. Risk of oral cancer in patients with graft-vs-host disease: a systematic review and meta-analysis. Oral Surg Oral Med Oral Pathol Oral Radiol. 2022 Jun;133(6):650–62.

Imanguli MM, Atkinson JC, Mitchell SA, Avila DN, Bishop RJ, Cowen EW, Datiles MB, Hakim FT, Kleiner DE, Krumlauf MC, Pavletic SZ. Salivary gland involvement in chronic graft-versus-host disease: prevalence, clinical significance, and recommendations for evaluation. Biol Blood Marrow Transplant. 2010 Oct;16(10):1362–9. Erratum in: Biol Blood Marrow Transplant. 2016 Jun;22(6):1147.

Johnson LB, Oh U, Rothen M, Sroussi HY, Dean DR, Lloid CM, Cintron K, Lee SJ, Cutler CS, Treister NS. A review of oral chronic graft-versus-host disease: considerations for dental hygiene practice. J Dent Hyg. 2022 Apr;96(2):6–17.

Mays JW, Fassil H, Edwards DA, Pavletic SZ, Bassim CW. Oral chronic graft-versus-host disease: current pathogenesis, therapy, and research. Oral Dis. 2013 May;19(4):327–46.

Pengpis N, Prueksrisakul T, Chanswangphuwana C. Clinical characteristics of oral chronic graft-versus-host disease according to the 2014 National Institutes of Health (USA) consensus criteria. Med Oral Patol Oral Cir Bucal. 2023 Mar 1;28(2):e167–73.

Shulman HM, Cardona DM, Greenson JK, Hingorani S, Horn T, Huber E, Kreft A, Longerich T, Morton T, Myerson D, Prieto VG, Rosenberg A, Treister N, Washington K, Ziemer M, Pavletic SZ, Lee SJ, Flowers ME, Schultz KR, Jagasia M, Martin PJ, Vogelsang GB, Kleiner DE. NIH Consensus development project on criteria for clinical trials in chronic graft-versus-host disease: II. The 2014 pathology working group report. Biol Blood Marrow Transplant. 2015 Apr;21(4):589–603.

Stolze J, Boor M, Hazenberg MD, Brand HS, Raber-Durlacher JE, Laheij AMGA. Oral health-related quality of life of patients with oral chronic graft-versus-host disease. Support Care Cancer. 2021 Nov;29(11):6353–60.

Chapter 14
Antimicrobial Photodynamic Therapy in the Treatment of Osteonecrosis Related to Radiotherapy or Medication

Aljomar José Vechiato Filho, Maria Cecília Querido de Oliveira, Letícia Lang, Ana Carolina Prado-Ribeiro, and Luiz Alcino Monteiro Gueiros

Treatment Definition

The antimicrobial photodynamic therapy (aPDT) has been recently suggested to conservatively treat ORN or MRONJ due to its promising anecdotal results. Considering that a wide range of bacteria units will colonize the surface of exposed necrotic bone in the oral cavity, ORN and MRONJ are frequently associated with acute infections and fistulas. Therefore, the potential efficacy of aPDT application may be explained by the microbial death and apoptosis process created because of a photooxidation reaction that occurs when a photosensitizing agent (PA) —e.g., methylene blue, toluidine blue, or malachite green—is irradiated with a luminous source at an appropriate resonant wavelength (red laser at 660 nm).

The physicochemical characteristics of PA allow them to penetrate the outer membrane of gram-negative bacteria. Then, the laser irradiation of such impregnated membrane results in an interesting physics phenomenon. Reactive oxygen specimens (ROS) are created into a quantic state named as singlet oxygen, which may be understood as ROS with electrons aligned. When this occurs, a high cytotoxic effect is induced, membrane cells are damage, and bacteria die.

The role of inflammation and infection in the prevalence, severity, and resolution of MRONJ and ORN disease is irrefutable. The presence of bacteria in exposed necrotic bone also contributes to disease severity, pain, and morbidity. Thus,

A. J. Vechiato Filho · M. C. Q. de Oliveira (✉) · A. C. Prado-Ribeiro
Dental Oncology Service, Insituto do Cancer do Estado de Sao Paulo (ICESP), University of São Paulo, São Paulo, SP, Brazil

L. Lang
Oncology and Radiotherapy Center of Londrina, Private Practice, Londrina, PR, Brazil

L. A. M. Gueiros
Clinical and Preventive Dentistry Department, Federal University of Pernambuco, Recife, PE, Brazil

A. R. Santos-Silva et al. (eds.), *Photobiomodulation Therapy in Oral Medicine*,
https://doi.org/10.1007/978-3-031-85048-6_14

although tooth extraction is the main cause of osteonecrosis of the jaws described in the literature, some studies have shown that the presence of infection carries more risk than the extraction itself.

In this sense, aPDT plays an important role in treating osteonecrosis of jaws since, by controlling the infection in and around the necrotic bone, this may be enough to induce the formation of bone sequestration, expelling the necrotic bone and leading to healing. Furthermore, photobiomodulation (PBM) improves the quality of the soft tissue around the necrotic bone, reducing inflammation and accelerating healing.

Another advantage to be considered is the possibility of decontaminating the necrotic bone itself with aPDT, as the penetration of the photosensitizer can lead to the effect of the therapy in deeper bone areas, which is not achieved with antibiotics or mouthwashes.

Despite the abovementioned features, literature is not clear for clinicians who search a clear-cut answer regarding the most appropriate aPDT protocol for MRONJ and ORN treatment. However, it may be suggested that aPDT is a useful tool, as follows:

1. First conservative option to solve the necrotic bone exposure, associated with antibiotic treatment.
2. Immediately after dental extraction(s) before sutures.
3. Immediately after cautions surgical removal of necrotic bone exposure (sequestrectomy).
4. Complementary therapy to be used in appointments between sessions for surgical approaches (cautions or not) until lesion is completely healed.

According to the pooled result of selected sources, aPDT was generally associated to antibiotic therapy, mainly for patients who developed acute infections (e.g., abscess and extra- and/or intraoral fistulas), or previously to dental extraction. Treating infections is necessary because purulent secretions will prevent the contact between PA and the surface of necrotic bone. Besides, newly extracted sockets with significant bleedings may have the same undesired situation.

However, it is noted that when introducing aPDT it is possible to use antibiotics for a shorter period, as local control of the infection will be achieved. Another indication described in case reports is the use of aPDT to minimize the risk of osteonecrosis in patients who need extractions but have already used antiresorptive drugs or have already received radiotherapy in the head and neck region.

The current literature suggests that PBM with a healing purpose may be performed or in the same clinical appointment for aPDT and in different days to aPDT to improve healing, control post-operatory symptoms, and optimize surgical results. It was not possible to suggest a unique protocol combining aPDT and PBM because the strategy used for aPDT and PBM sessions diverged significantly among cases reported in the same article and in selected studies. Probably, the explanation for such finding is that everyone showed a different severity of infection and symptoms. However, it may be assumed that aPDT allows the clinicians to empirically combine both therapies (aPDT and PBM), while there are no scientific based protocols

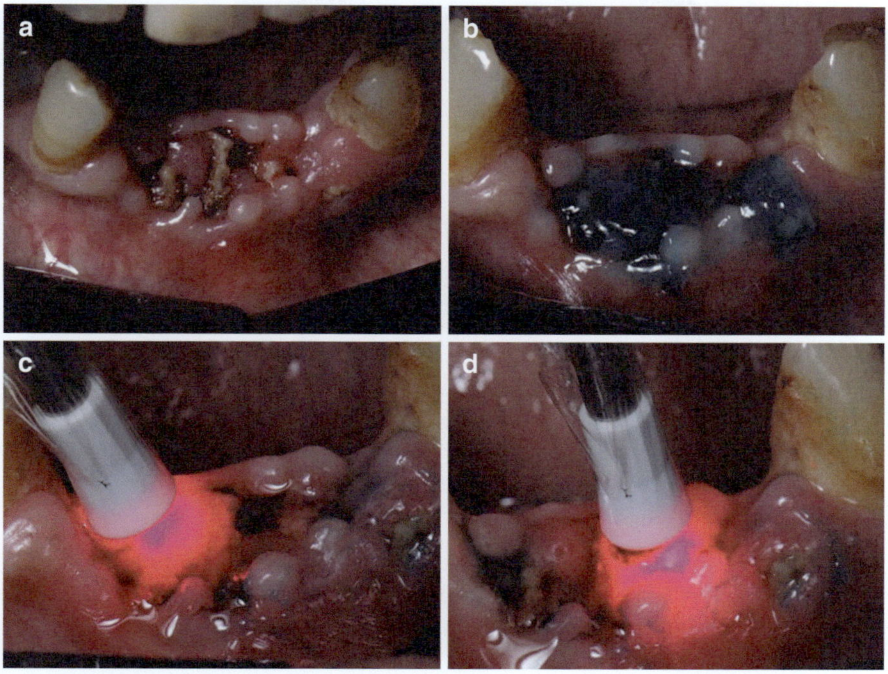

Fig. 14.1 (**a**) Stage 2 MRONJ in the anterior mandible. (**b**) Methylene blue 0.01% gel applied to the exposed necrotic bone for 5 min. (**c**, **d**) Red laser (660 nm) irradiation to the exposed bone

available in literature. As a suggestion, the strategy used by professionals should be based on the clinical aspect of the wound and on patient's symptoms. Figure 14.1 shows aPDT protocol in the treatment of MRONJ.

Diagnostic Criteria to Use aPDT

- Clinical evaluation (necrotic bone exposure associated or not to acute infection; intraoral and extraoral fistula).
- Possibility to conservatively treat MRONJ or ORN (elective cases).

Treatment

It is generally based on antiseptics and/or antibiotics, cautious debridement or sequestrectomies of exposed necrotic bone, the drug combination of pentoxyphilin–tocopherol (PENTO) or pentoxifylline–tocopherol–clodronate (PENTOCLO), hyperbaric oxygenation, and extensive surgical resections with or without reconstruction.

Figure 14.2 illustrates a case of ORN treated with surgical approach, antibiotic therapy, PENTO, and aPDT. However, disadvantages of the previously mentioned therapies “turn a light” on aPDT. Differently from such medication and surgical treatments (cautions or not), aPDT seems to be a very interesting tool because:

1. It is a noninvasive therapy.
2. It may be associated with PBM. Thus, it not only promotes microbial disinfection but also may induce tissue repair through all biostimulation features induced by laser irradiation.
3. There is no scientific evidence that suggests potential side effects or microbial resistance, and then aPDT can be repeated as many times as necessary.
4. It is possible to administer aPDT with an optical fiber to necrotic bone through a fistula, thus enabling the treatment of infection without surgical access.
5. aPDT is effective in combating other microorganisms commonly associated with necrotic bone, such as fungus.
6. It is a therapy that can be used in patients undergoing cancer treatment, who are often not eligible for surgical procedures.

It is important to properly clean the necrotic bone before performing aPDT to remove the biofilm. If there is blood or saliva, the PA must be replaced, as it may be

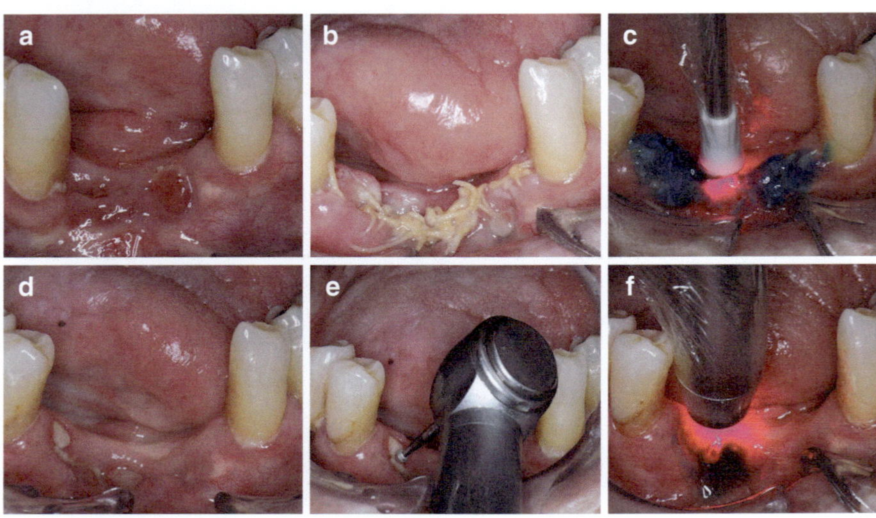

Fig. 14.2 Stage 2 ORN of the anterior mandible. (**a**) Patient underwent antibiotic therapy with amoxicillin/clavulanic acid for 14 days and metronidazole for 7 days. After completion of antibiotic therapy, the patient started the PENTO protocol. (**b**) Postoperative of 7 days after surgical approach (local debridement). (**c**) First session of aPDT, using PA (methylene blue 0.01% gel) and red laser (660 nm), 9 J, irradiated on the surgical wound. The patient was treated with weekly aPDT sessions with good progression. (**d**) Bone exposure persisted after 5 aPDT sessions and 45 days of PENTO protocol. (**e**) Osteoplasty with dental diamond bur. (**f**) aPDT sessions were performed three times a week with PA (methylene blue 0.01% gel for 5 min) and red laser (660 nm) irradiation on the exposed bone

diluted, and its concentration reduced. The choice of PA concentration must consider the presence of these competitors, which can cause its dilution. The suggestion of 0.01% methylene blue made for aPDT in osteonecrosis of the jaw considers the control of competitors (as blood and saliva). Relative isolation with cotton rollers is recommended.

Table 14.1 displays the summary of all information described in current literature to provide some basic guidelines that is supposed to drive professionals toward total healing in necrotic bone exposed lesions, associated or not with surgical treatments or other therapies. Besides, Table 14.1 complies the clinical expertise of the authors herein listed in the current chapter.

Table 14.1 Antimicrobial photodynamic therapy parameters suggested for treating medication-related osteonecrosis of the jaw and osteoradionecrosis

Wavelength (nm)		Red: 660
Power (mW)		100
Radiant energy (J)		9/point
Fluence (J/cm^2)		9
Photonic fluence	($p.J/cm^2$)	13.5
	(Einstein)	3
Exposure time (s/point)		90
Spot location		Exposed bone lesion Within dental socket, immediately after the tooth extraction[a] Into intraoral and extraoral fistula (with an optical fiber)
Treatment days		Prevention: Apply PA (e.g., 0.01% methylene blue) during 5 min and irradiate with red laser immediately after the tooth extraction within the dental socket or sequestrectomy. At first, there is no need to extend sessions[b] Treatment: Apply PA (e.g., 0.01% methylene blue) during 5 min and irradiate with red laser. Consider performing aPDT once a week[c]

[a]Selected studies recommend 500 mg Amoxicillin or 400 mg Ampicillin or 300 mg Clindamycin orally, based on previous history of drug allergy, 24 h preoperative and continued for 7 days post-operation

[b]Clinical appointments for aPDT before dental procedures may be interesting to improve decontamination of surface of exposed bone. Suggestion: 5 aPDT sessions

[c]There is no recommendation for treatment duration. Patient's symptoms may demand modifications to this strategy. Therefore, consider repeating until positive response since there is no scientific evidence contraindicating PBM continuity. However, surgical debridement is encouraged if the MRONJ/ORN area is increasing. PBM may be associated to enhance the postoperatory recovery

Treatment (aPDT May Be Associated with)

- *Systemic Pharmacological Treatment* (see ORN and MRONJ chapters for more info).
  - Analgesics.
  - Antibiotic therapy.
  - Pentoxyphilin–tocopherol (PENTO) or pentoxifylline–tocopherol–clodronate (PENTOCLO) combinations.
- *Topical Pharmacological Treatment.*
  - Oral antibacterial mouth rinse.
- *Surgical treatment.*
  - Cautious debridement or sequestrectomies of exposed necrotic bone.
  - Extensive surgical resections with or without reconstruction.
- *Photobiomodulation* (see MRONJ and ORN chapters for more info).

Further Reading

Campos L, Martins F, Tateno RY, Sendyk WR, Palma LF. Antimicrobial photodynamic therapy using optical fiber for oral fistula resulting from mandibular osteoradionecrosis. Photodiagn Photodyn Ther. 2021;34:102247.

Ribeiro GH, Minamisako MC, Rath IBDS, Santos AMB, Simões A, Pereira KCR, Grando LJ. Osteoradionecrosis of the jaws: case series treated with adjuvant low-level laser therapy and antimicrobial photodynamic therapy. J Appl Oral Sci. 2018;26:e20170172.

Schussel JL, de Araújo AMM, Ballardin BS, Torres-Pereira CC. Antimicrobial photodynamic therapy as a treatment option for inoperable cases of medication-related osteonecrosis of the jaws. Photodiagn Photodyn Ther. 2022;39:102947.

Tartaroti NC, Marques MM, Naclério-Homem MDG, Migliorati CA, Zindel Deboni MC. Antimicrobial photodynamic and photobiomodulation adjuvant therapies for prevention and treatment of medication-related osteonecrosis of the jaws: case series and long-term follow-up. Photodiagn Photodyn Ther. 2020;29:101651.

Part III
Oral Medicine

Oral medicine is the specialty that aims to integrate dentistry and medicine. The practice of oral medicine specialists focuses on the diagnosis and nonsurgical management of diseases and conditions of the oral and maxillofacial areas. Oral diseases and conditions are commonly managed by the oral medicine specialist using medical therapy with various topical and systemic medications. Although several protocols exist for the management of a myriad of common orofacial disorders, new diseases and the use of new systemic medications for the treatment of medical problems often represent a management challenge for the oral medicine specialist. Many diseases affecting the oral cavity have an inflammatory basis, may become superinfected, and may be refractory to the common therapies. Therefore, there is a constant search for new therapies and protocols to manage oral diseases.

It has been demonstrated that PBM is effective in preventing and treating various conditions common in oral medicine, including mucocutaneous inflammatory conditions, chronic diseases, infections, and neuropathic disorders. PBMT has proven to be an effective, nondrug, and noninvasive method for alleviating symptoms or achieving complete resolution of various oral diseases, either as a stand-alone or as an adjunct therapy.

The following chapters will present recommended protocols for treating common oral diseases with PBM and/or antimicrobial photodynamic therapy, aiming to provide an alternative, effective, and cost-beneficial method for clinicians and their patients.

Further Reading

Kalhori KAM, Vahdatinia F, Jamalpour MR, Vescovi P, Fornaini C, Merigo E, Fekrazad R. Photobiomodulation in oral medicine. Photobiomodul Photomed Laser Surg. 2019 Dec;37(12):837–61.

Pandeshwar P, Roa MD, Das R, Shastry SP, Kaul R, Srinivasreddy MB. Photobiomodulation in oral medicine: a review. J Investig Clin Dent. 2016 May;7(2):114–26.

Chapter 15
Recurrent Aphthous Stomatitis

Eliete Neves Silva Guerra, Juliana Amorim dos Santos, César Rivera, Karen Patricia Domínguez Gallagher, Eduardo David Piemonte, and Gloria Jeanethe Alvarez Gómez

Disease Definition

Recurrent aphthous stomatitis (RAS) is an inflammatory ulcer of unknown etiology that affects mainly the nonkeratinized oral mucosa. It is the most common oral mucosal disease worldwide presenting incidences up to 25% depending on the geographical region. A painful round- or oval-shaped ulcer with an erythematous halo covered by a fibrin layer that heals spontaneously characterizes the condition. In the literature, aphthae are divided into three types: minor aphthous (2–10 mm in diameter), which is the most common, major aphthous (also called periadenitis mucosa necrotica recurrens, >10 mm in diameter, with resultant scarring), and herpetiform ulceration (multiple small ulcers). The disease causes severe discomfort for the patient due to pain, leading to difficulties in eating, drinking, speaking, chewing, swallowing, and maintaining oral hygiene. The impact on quality of life is largely explained by the number and size of the lesions.

E. N. S. Guerra (✉) · J. Amorim dos Santos
Faculty of Health Sciences, Laboratory of Oral Histopathology, University of Brasília, Brasília, DF, Brazil
e-mail: elieteneves@unb.br

C. Rivera
Faculty of Dentistry, Department of Stomatology, Laboratory of Oral and Maxillofacial Histopathology, University of Talca, Talca, Chile

K. P. D. Gallagher
School of Dentistry, National University of Asunción, Asunción, Paraguay

E. D. Piemonte
Oral Medicine Department "A", Dentistry College, National University of Córdoba, Córdoba, Argentina

G. J. A. Gómez
School of Dentistry, University of Antioquia, Medellín, Colombia

A. R. Santos-Silva et al. (eds.), *Photobiomodulation Therapy in Oral Medicine*,
https://doi.org/10.1007/978-3-031-85048-6_15

Despite this disease's frequency, the etiopathogenesis of RAS still needs to be fully understood, which would explain why RAS is still common today. However, recent studies on the etiology and pathogenesis include different inflammatory reactions, and there are some suggested predisposing factors, such as a family history of aphthous lesions or systemic disorders like vitamin and other dietary deficits (e.g., folic acid, iron, zinc, vitamin B_1, B_2, B_6, and B_{12}) with or without underlying gastrointestinal condition (e.g., Crohn's disease, celiac disease, or ulcerative rectocolitis), endocrine imbalance (e.g., menarche, menstruation, and menopause), HIV infection, stress, trauma, and allergies. Current investigations suggest that gene polymorphisms might be associated with RAS pathogenesis. Most risk factors for the disease are single nucleotide polymorphisms in genes associated with immune system function (such as TLR4, MMP9, E-selectin, IL-1 beta, and TNF-alpha). These genetic polymorphisms are nonmodifiable risk factors, suggesting that susceptibility to RAS is, at least partially, inherited, and these factors cannot be altered.

Among the differential diagnoses of RAS, minor lesions can be mentioned, such as acute traumatic ulcers, others that require specific treatments, such as herpes lesions or Behçet's disease, and even diseases that put the patient's life at risk, such as cyclic neutropenia or autoimmune blistering diseases. It is imperative that an accurate diagnosis be obtained to select the optimal treatment.

Diagnosis

- Clinical evaluation.

Treatment

Topical and systemic modalities are available to treat RAS. Not surprisingly, the characteristics of RAS symptoms described above require therapeutic strategies that aim to promote immediate pain alleviation and, ideally, decrease the frequency or even stop the onset of acute phases. Systemic medication may be used following ineffective topical treatment. However, the literature affirms that clinicians should not disregard the adverse effects of systemic medications because of their tangible positive effects. A Cochrane review showed that the effect of systemic medication does not outweigh the adverse effects of the drugs used. Therefore, clinicians may prefer therapies that minimize the risk of adverse events. The pharmacological agents proposed for topical treatment include anti-inflammatory drugs, antiseptics, antibiotics, anesthetics, corticosteroids, and plant-derived biomolecules. Different wavelengths of lasers have been demonstrated satisfactory effects on cell metabolism, inflammatory modulation, edema reduction, tissue regeneration, healing time, and pain relief.

Current evidence shows that photobiomodulation (PBM) for RAS should have better results when low doses of energy density (≈ 2 J/cm^2) (Fig. 15.1) are used than

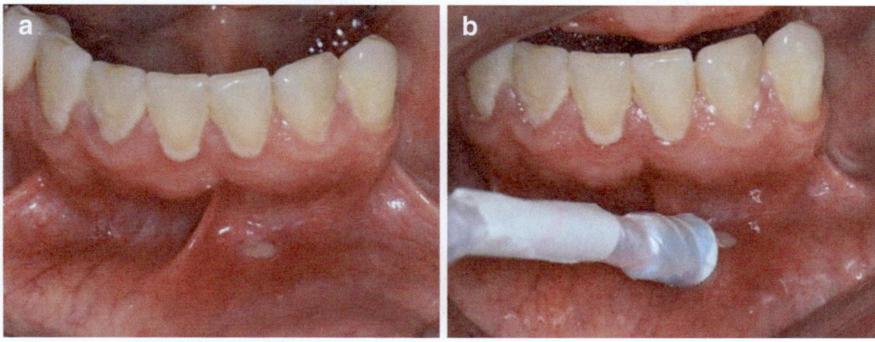

Fig. 15.1 (**a**) RAS ulcer on the labial vestibule of the mandible. (**b**) NIR laser (2 J) being applied to the ulcer

Table 15.1 Photobiomodulation parameters suggested for treating recurrent aphthous stomatitis

Wavelength (nm)		Red: 660	NIR: 810
Power (mW)		100	
Radiant energy (J)		2/point	
Fluence (J/cm^2)		2	
Photonic fluence	($p.J/cm^2$)	≈ 3.8	≈ 3
	(Einstein)	≈ 0.8	≈ 0.6
Exposure time (s/point)		20	
Spot location		One single central point on each aphthous lesion	
Treatment days		Wound healing: a single session[a] Pain relief: Once a day for two days	

[a]NIR wavelength is recommended for wound healing

higher doses because of a possible effect suppressive or inhibitory effect (e.g., ≥ 16 J/cm^2) is used. However, the parameters for PBM with diode lasers are very heterogeneous. Therefore, the parameters of Table 15.1 should be carefully considered by clinicians when treating RAS.

Treatment

- *Systemic Pharmacological Treatment.*
  - Analgesics and anti-inflammatory agents.
- *Topical Pharmacological Treatment.*
  - Topical or intra-lesion corticosteroids.
  - Anesthetics topical agents.
  - Cyanoacrylate-based protective bio adhesives (cyanoacrylate).
  - Antiseptic or anti-inflammatory therapies.
- *Photobiomodulation.*

Further Reading

Albrektson M, Hedström L, Bergh H. Recurrent aphthous stomatitis and pain management with low-level laser therapy: a randomized controlled trial. Oral Surg Oral Med Oral Pathol Oral Radiol. 2014;117:590–4.

Amorim Dos Santos J, Normando AGC, de Toledo IP, Melo G, De Luca CG, Santos-Silva AR, Guerra ENS. Laser therapy for recurrent aphthous stomatitis: an overview. Clin Oral Investig. 2020 Jan;24(1):37–45.

Brocklehurst P, Tickle M, Glenny AM, Lewis MA, Pemberton MN, Taylor J, Walsh T, Riley P, Yates JM. Systemic interventions for recurrent aphthous stomatitis (mouth ulcers). Cochrane Database Syst Rev. 2012 Sep 12;9:CD005411.

Edgar NR, Saleh D, Miller RA. Recurrent Aphthous stomatitis: a review. J Clin Aesthet Dermatol. 2017 Mar;10(3):26–36.

Gaizeh Al-Hallak MA, Chalhoub K, Hsaian JA, Aljoujou AA. Efficacy of photobiomodulation therapy in recurrent herpes labialis management: a randomized controlled trial. Clin Oral Investig. 2024 Feb 20;28(2):157.

Hernández-Olivos R, Muñoz M, Núñez E, Camargo-Ayala PA, Garcia-Huidobro J, Pereira A, Nachtigall FM, Santos LS, Rivera C. Salivary proteome of aphthous stomatitis reveals the participation of vitamin metabolism, nutrients, and bacteria. Sci Rep. 2021 Aug 2;11(1):15646.

Monteiro MM, Amorim Dos Santos J, Paiva Barbosa V, Rezende TMB, Guerra ENS. Photobiomodulation effects on fibroblasts and keratinocytes after ionizing radiation and bacterial stimulus. Arch Oral Biol. 2024 Mar;159:105874.

Parra-Moreno FJ, Egido-Moreno S, Schemel-Suárez M, González-Navarro B, Estrugo-Devesa A, López-López J. Treatment of recurrent aphthous stomatitis: a systematic review. Med Oral Patol Oral Cir Bucal. 2023 Jan 1;28(1):e87–98.

Rivera C, Muñoz-Pastén M, Núñez-Muñoz E, Hernández-Olivos R. Recurrent Aphthous stomatitis affects quality of life. A case-control study. Clin Cosmet Investig. Dent. 2022 Jul 26;14:217–23.

Rivera C. Essentials of recurrent aphthous stomatitis. Biomed Rep. 2019 Aug;11(2):47–50.

Rocca JP, Zhao M, Fornaini C, Tan L, Zhao Z, Merigo E. Effect of laser irradiation on aphthae pain management: a four different wavelengths comparison. J Photochem Photobiol B. 2018 Dec;189:1–4.

Suter VGA, Sjölund S, Bornstein MM. Effect of laser on pain relief and wound healing of recurrent aphthous stomatitis: a systematic review. Lasers Med Sci. 2017;32:953–63.

Tezel A, Kara C, Balkaya V, Orbak R. An evaluation of different treatments for recurrent aphthous stomatitis and patient perceptions: Nd:YAG laser versus medication. Photomed Laser Surg. 2009 Feb;27(1):101–6.

Chapter 16
Recurrent Herpes Labialis

Aljomar José Vechiato Filho, Maria Cecília Querido de Oliveira, Ana Carolina Prado Ribeiro, Diego Tetzner Fernandes, Leonor Victória González Pérez, and Márcio Diniz-Freitas

Disease Definition

Recurrent herpes labialis (RHL) is an infection caused by herpes simplex virus type 1 (HSV-1). The incidence of this infection is approximately 1.6 per 1000 patients, with a prevalence of 2.5 per 1000 patients per year. These figures may vary between different countries and communities. The World Health Organization estimates that 3.7 billion people under the age of 50 (67%) worldwide are infected with the virus, with one-third of them experiencing at least one relapse per year.

Most primary infections are transmitted directly through contact with an infected lesion or body fluids. HSV-1 binds to specific cell surface receptors and disrupts the host cell nucleus by replicating the viral genome. The host may exhibit signs and symptoms, including multiple oral vesicles, fever, malaise, chills, fatigue, nausea, loss of appetite, lethargy, irritability, and headache, which may last 10–14 days.

Following the initial infection, HSV-1 penetrates the sensory nerve endings and is transported by retrograde axonal pathway to neuronal cell bodies, where a more restricted replication cycle occurs. This constitutes a latent infection of these

A. J. Vechiato Filho · M. C. Q. de Oliveira · A. C. P. Ribeiro
Dental Oncology Service, São Paulo State Cancer Institute, University of São Paulo Medical School, São Paulo, SP, Brazil

D. T. Fernandes (✉)
Private Practice, Limeira, SP, Brazil

L. V. G. Pérez
University of Antioquia, Medellín, Colombia

Oral Diagnosis Department, Piracicaba Dental School, University of Campinas, Piracicaba, SP, Brazil

M. Diniz-Freitas
Medical-Surgical Dentistry Research Group, Health Research Institute of Santiago de Compostela, University of Santiago de Compostela, Santiago de Compostela, Spain

A. R. Santos-Silva et al. (eds.), *Photobiomodulation Therapy in Oral Medicine*,
https://doi.org/10.1007/978-3-031-85048-6_16

neurons, which remain dormant until reactivation occurs. The trigeminal ganglion is the main site of latency, where the virus remains present throughout life.

Although the first episode of herpes simplex infection is the more intense, recurrence can be precipitated by a multitude of factors, including psychological distress, surgical trauma, hormonal fluctuations in women, hyperthermia, or infectious diseases. Additionally, ultraviolet radiation, corticosteroids, and other pharmaceutical agents can also contribute to the development of persistent episodes. Such recurrences often have profound psychosocial implications for patients.

During recurrence, the virus reactivates and migrates through the sensory nerves to the basal skin and mucosal cells of the lips and perioral area, where it replicates and activates immune reactions that initiate a clinical episode. This episode typically takes between 7 and 10 days to unfold, with the following phases:

- Prodromal.
  This phase is present in 60% of patients and lasts for up to 24 h. It is characterized by pain, burning, itching, or tingling at the site where the lesions will appear. Clinically, erythema may be observed.
- Vesicles and pustules.
  These phases last several hours and involve the rupture of vesicles and pustules, respectively. During this phase, the vesicles and pustules contain active infectious viruses.
- Ulcers.
  This phase lasts a few hours and is marked by the formation of ulcers, which are covered with a yellowish liquid (fibrin). In some cases, the ulcers may be accompanied by surrounding erythema.
- Crusting.
  This phase begins with the formation of a soft crust, which is replaced by a hard crust over the course of 5–6 days.
- Healing.
  This phase generally results in the absence of scarring.

Diagnosis

- Clinical evaluation (recurrent blistering).
- PCR test, viral culture, or electron microscopy.
- Exfoliative cytology.
- Serological test (antibodies).

Treatment

The conventional treatment for RHL relies on topical or systemic antiviral agents (such as acyclovir, valacyclovir, and famciclovir). However, when initiated during the prodromal or initial stages (before vesicle formation), these medications primarily offer symptomatic relief since their mechanism targets viral replication. Consequently, only a limited number of patients experience significant benefits from these medications. Moreover, these drugs also do not have the potential to cure the latent infection and only show a limited reduction in lesions healing time.

Clinicians have been exploring effective treatments to prevent RHL recurrence because of all the disease features discussed above. Some studies have shown that antiviral drugs may prevent recurrence when used prophylactically. However, oral bioavailability is low following oral administration, necessitating multiple doses per day. This frequent dosing schedule can be burdensome for patients to maintain, often leading to poor adherence to the prescribed regimen. Additionally, nephrotoxicity may limit their intake, mainly for patients with kidney disease. Therefore, photobiomodulation (PBM) has been suggested by some clinical trials as an effective alternative that can significantly shorten the RHL episodes, reduce its signs and symptoms, and decrease disease recurrence with the benefit of a side effect-free therapy.

In this context, some case reports have described promising results when combining antimicrobial photodynamic therapy (aPDT) with PBM, and however, up to date, no clinical trials to have confirmed the efficacy of this combination. Methylene blue has been used in all these case reports as the photosensitizing agent (PA) associated with low-level lasers with a wavelength of 660 nm as the light source. Figure 16.1 illustrates a case of aPDT for RHL in the perioral region, using the suggested PBM parameters presented in Table 16.1.

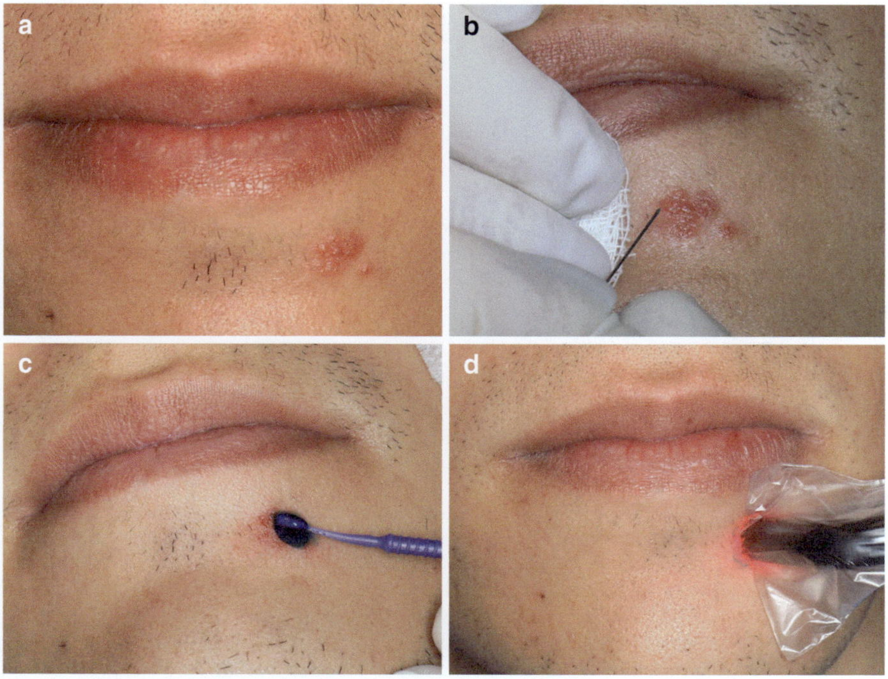

Fig. 16.1 aPDT for RHL in the perioral region. (**a**) Signs of RHL (vesicle phase) in the perioral region. (**b**) Vesicles drainage by using needle. (**c**) Photosensitizing agent (PA) application (methylene blue 0.01%) (**d**) Red laser (660 nm) for 20 s

Table 16.1 Photobiomodulation parameters suggested for treating recurrent herpes labialis

Wavelength (nm)		Red: 660	NIR: 810
Power (mW)		100	
Radiant energy (J)		2/point	
Fluence (J/cm^2)		2	
Photonic fluence	(p.J/cm^2)	≈ 3.8	≈ 3
	(Einstein)	≈ 0.8	≈ 0.6
Exposure time (s/point)		20	
Spot location		Curative (Red): on lesion and surroundings + aPDT (Vesicles phase–vesicles drainage by using a needle followed by aPDT. Crust phase–PBM) Preventive (NIR): lips and perioral region[a]	
Treatment days		Curative (Red): twice weekly sessions, alternate days until complete healing Preventive (NIR): five sessions with 48 h interval between them at 6 and 12 months after the curative sessions[a]	

[a]Performed to minimize recurrence

The use of aPDT is indicated in the vesicle phase (after drainage of the vesicle content with a sterile needle or a high-power laser), while PBM can be used in other phases of manifestation, such as the latent, prodromal, and crust phases. Thus, PBM is assumed to be not only effective for preventing RHL recurrence but also to improve healing and reducing symptoms.

Treatment

- *Systemic Pharmacological Treatment.*
  - Antiviral drugs (acyclovir, valacyclovir, and famciclovir).
- *Topical Pharmacological Treatment.*
  - Antiviral drug (acyclovir or penciclovir).
- *Photobiomodulation.*

Further Reading

Arduino PG, Porter SR. Herpes Simplex Virus Type 1 infection: overview on relevant clinico-pathological features. J Oral Pathol Med. 2008 Feb;37(2):107–21.

Eduardo CP, Bezinelli LM, Eduardo FP, Graça Lopes RM, Ramalho KM, Bello-Silva MS, Esteves-Oliveira M. Prevention of recurrent herpes labialis outbreaks through low-intensity laser therapy: a clinical protocol with 3-year follow-up. Lasers Med Sci. 2012;27:1077–83.

Gopinath D, Koe KH, Maharajan MK, Panda S. A comprehensive overview of epidemiology, pathogenesis and the management of herpes labialis. Viruses. 2023;15:225.

James C, Harfouche M, Welton NJ, Turner KM, Abu-Raddad LJ, Gottlieb SL, Looker KJ. Herpes simplex virus: global infection prevalence and incidence estimates, 2016. Bull World Health Organ. 2020 May 1;98(5):315–29.

Khalil M, Hamadah O. Association of photodynamic therapy and photobiomodulation as a promising treatment of herpes labialis: a systematic review. Photobiomodul Photomed Laser Surg. 2022;40:299–307.

Petti S, Lodi G. The controversial natural history of oral herpes simplex virus type 1 infection. Oral Dis. 2019 Nov;25(8):1850–65.

Zanella PA, Onuchic LF, Watanabe EH, Azevedo LH, Aranha ACC, Ramalho KM, Eduardo CP. Photobiomodulation for preventive therapy of recurrent herpes labialis: a 2-year in vivo randomized controlled study. Photobiomodul Photomed Laser Surg. 2022;40:682–90.

Chapter 17
Lichen Planus

Rafael Tomaz Gomes, Luiz Alcino Monteiro Gueiros, Javier I. Giménez, Verónica E. Flück, Ángeles Castrillo, Claudia A. Giacco, Jairo Robledo-Sierra, and Joel B. Epstein

Disease Definition

Oral lichen planus (OLP) is a relatively common chronic mucocutaneous disorder that affects nearly 1% of the global population. Although the exact etiopathogenesis of OLP is still unclear, current evidence supports an inflammatory cell-mediated immune response to an unknown trigger. It usually affects individuals between the ages of 30 and 65 years, with a slight female predisposition. The buccal mucosa is the most affected site, followed by the tongue and gingiva. However, any site of the oral cavity can be affected. Clinically, OLP is classified as reticular, papular, plaque-type, bullous, atrophic, and erosive. Reticular OLP is the most common form, and it is mostly asymptomatic, requiring no treatment. In contrast, atrophic and erosive forms usually present erythematous, ulcerative areas causing symptoms, ranging from mild burning sensation to severe pain, interfering with eating and speaking.

R. T. Gomes
Department of Dermatology, Federal University of São Paulo, São Paulo, SP, Brazil

L. A. M. Gueiros
Clinical and Preventive Dentistry Department, Federal University of Pernambuco, Recife, PE, Brazil

J. I. Giménez · V. E. Flück · Á. Castrillo · C. A. Giacco
Stomatology Service, Oncology Hospital of Buenos Aires Marie Curie, Buenos Aires, Argentina

J. Robledo-Sierra
CES University, Medellín, Colombia

J. B. Epstein (✉)
Cedars-Sinai Health System, Los Angeles, CA, USA

City of Hope National Medical Center, Duarte, CA, USA
e-mail: jepstein@coh.org

A. R. Santos-Silva et al. (eds.), *Photobiomodulation Therapy in Oral Medicine*,
https://doi.org/10.1007/978-3-031-85048-6_17

These symptoms greatly affect the patients' s quality of life, which requires medical intervention.

Skin manifestations can be associated with OLP and are classically presented as flat topped, purple, polygonal, pruritic papules on the volar aspect of wrists and forearms, ankles, lower legs, and lumbosacral spine.

Biopsy is mandatory for the diagnosis of OLP. Histopathologically, an infiltration of T lymphocytes destroying the basal stratum, is seen, which causes white striae and, sometimes, erosions or ulcers. Direct immunofluorescence can assist the pathologist in confirming the diagnosis for refractory cases. Clinical–histopathological correlation is important for a definitive diagnosis to be established.

Diagnosis

- Clinical evaluation
- Biopsy (H&E stain and immunofluorescence)

Treatment

Therapeutic methods such as topical and systemic corticosteroids are frequently used. However, if used chronically as the sole option to treat OLP, these immunosuppressive agents may induce opportunistic infections, adrenal gland impairment, and mucosal atrophy. Besides, some cases may become refractory to such a strategy with prolonged usage. Other management alternatives include antimalarials, calcineurin inhibitors, mTOR inhibitors, and non-pharmacological interventions such as photobiomodulation (PBM) and laser surgery.

In recent years, the interest in PBM as an alternative modality for treating OLP has progressively increased. A head-to-head randomized controlled trial (RCT) showed a similar efficacy between PBM and topical clobetasol, a well-studied and common treatment. This fact may be explained by the laser irradiance that will reduce clinical signs and symptoms because of the differentiation and migration of fibroblasts, increased proliferation, enhancement of cellular activity, and the reduction of inflammation through an immunomodulation action (boost of mast cell function, which releases more leucocytes into oral tissues).

Besides, the safety and the absence of adverse effects of PBM overcome the conventional methods. Furthermore, some studies show that patients treated with PBM have more prolonged times without recurrence of OLP lesions than when corticosteroids were employed. However, the methods substantially varied among studies though there is a high level of evidence available in the literature. Finally, it is worth mentioning that no studies compared both methods even though some authors suggest that this combination should not be disregarded for those patients

Table 17.1 Photobiomodulation parameters suggested for treating oral lichen planus[a]

Wavelength (nm)		Red: 660	NIR: 808–970
Power (mW)		40–100	100–300
Radiant energy (J)		1/point	2–3/point
Fluence (J/cm^2)		1	3
Photonic fluence	(p.J/cm^2)	≈ 1.9	≈ 3.9–4.5
	(Einstein)	≈ 0.4	≈ 0.8–1
Exposure time (s/point)		20	
Spot location		3–4 points above and around each lesion/area	
Treatment days		Twice a week for 4–6 weeks	

[a]Greater results may occur when PBM is associated with topical corticosteroids

with significant painful lesions. It is assumed that corticosteroids may boost the PBM effect in those scenarios. Table 17.1 shows the PBM parameters for OLP.

Treatment

- *Systemic Pharmacological Treatment*
  - Analgesics and anti-inflammatory drugs
    It is recommended to discuss with the patient's dermatologist the prescription of opioids to ensure the most suitable analgesic protocol. Physicians usually consider all steps of pain management scale when prescribing analgesics.
  - Calcineurin inhibitors
  - mammalian target of rapamycin (mTOR) inhibitors
  - Immunobiologics/ Janus kinases/signal transducer (JAK/STR) signaling pathway inhibitors
- *Topical Pharmacological Treatment*
  - Anesthetics and analgesic (sprays, mouthwashes, and gels)
  - Corticosteroids (mouthwashes and gels)
  - Immunomodulators (e.g., calcineurin inhibitors, tacrolimus, and pimecrolimus)
- *Laser Surgery*
  CO_2 laser ablation has also shown promising results in the management of OLP, reducing the symptoms and promoting a prolonged lesion-free period.
- *Photobiomodulation*

Further Reading

Akram Z, Abduljabbar T, Vohra F, Javed F. Efficacy of low-level laser therapy compared to steroid therapy in the treatment of oral lichen planus: a systematic review. J Oral Pathol Med. 2018;47:11–7.

Al-Maweri SA, Kalakonda B, Al-Soneidar WA, Al-Shamiri HM, Alakhali MS, Alaizari N. Efficacy of low-level laser therapy in management of symptomatic oral lichen planus: a systematic review. Lasers Med Sci. 2017;32:1429–37.

Boch K, Langan EA, Kridin K, Zillikens D, Ludwig RJ, Bieber K. Lichen planus. Front Med (Lausanne). 2021 Nov 1;8:737813.

El-Howati A, Thornhill MH, Colley HE, Murdoch C. Immune mechanisms in oral lichen planus. Oral Dis. 2023 May;29(4):1400–15.

González-Moles MÁ, Warnakulasuriya S, González-Ruiz I, González-Ruiz L, Ayén Á, Lenouvel D, Ruiz-Ávila I, Ramos-García P. Worldwide prevalence of oral lichen planus: a systematic review and meta-analysis. Oral Dis. 2021 May;27(4):813–28.

Sandhu S, Klein BA, Al-Hadlaq M, Chirravur P, Bajonaid A, Xu Y, Intini R, Hussein M, Vacharotayangul P, Sroussi H, Treister N, Sonis S. Oral lichen planus: comparative efficacy and treatment costs-a systematic review. BMC Oral Health. 2022 May 6;22(1):161.

Chapter 18
Pemphigus Vulgaris

Daniela Adorno Farias, Josefina Martínez-Ramírez, Wilfredo Alejandro González-Arriagada, and Pablo Agustin Vargas

Disease Definition

Pemphigus vulgaris (PV) is the most common variant of pemphigus, a systemic bullous autoimmune disease characterized by acantholysis due to autoantibodies against desmoglein 1 and 3. Both genders are affected, but PV commits women slightly more frequently on their fourth and sixth decades of life. Although PV is a rare condition with an incidence of up to 16 cases per million per year worldwide, it commonly presents with painful blisters and erosions on the skin and mucous membranes, particularly in the oral cavity associated with dysphagia and weight loss. Studies have demonstrated that the manifestations on the oral mucosa are the first signs of such autoimmune disorder, preceding other manifestations.

Other symptoms include hoarseness, dysphagia, odynophagia, throat pain, and bleeding, reflecting the involvement of the gastrointestinal tract, especially the oral cavity and esophagus. In severe cases, PV can manifest as extensive skin and mucosal lesions resembling Stevens–Johnson syndrome/toxic epidermal necrolysis. Additionally, PV can rarely occur in patients with human immunodeficiency virus (HIV), leading to widespread skin lesions, blisters, denuded areas, and pruritic crusts, which can progress rapidly and be life-threatening.

D. A. Farias
Oral Medicine and Pathology Department, School of Dentistry, University of Chile, Santiago, Chile

J. Martínez-Ramírez · P. A. Vargas (✉)
Oral Diagnosis Department, Piracicaba Dental School, University of Campinas, Piracicaba, SP, Brazil
e-mail: pavargas@fop.unicamp.br

W. A. González-Arriagada
Faculty of Dentistry, University of Los Andes, Santiago, Chile

A. R. Santos-Silva et al. (eds.), *Photobiomodulation Therapy in Oral Medicine*,
https://doi.org/10.1007/978-3-031-85048-6_18

The definitive diagnosis of PV is achieved by analysis of a perilesional tissue biopsy under histopathological examination, direct immunofluorescence (DIF), or indirect immunofluorescence. The criterion for histopathological diagnosis of PV is the presence of acantholysis with an inflammatory infiltration and presence of Tzank cells, while the DIF reveals intercellular accumulation of IgG against Dsg1 and/or Dsg3.

Diagnosis

- Clinical evaluation
- Biopsy (histopathological examination, direct immunofluorescence, or indirect immunofluorescence)

Treatment

The goal of PV treatment is to induce remission of signs and symptoms and prevent the formation of new lesions until the end of systemic treatment. To date, there has been no international consensus regarding the treatment strategy of PV. Systemic steroids are the gold standard treatment for this condition. However, PV is not rarely associated with ulcers that resist to complete healing (phenomenon named as "recalcitrant lesions" in published articles), and their management will bring the patients into a significant undesired situation of prolonged corticosteroid use leading to various adverse effects.

In this context, photobiomodulation (PBM) has been suggested to be combined with conventional therapies, especially in PV patients who do not show significant responses to corticosteroids or for those individuals with recalcitrant ulcers. However, there are no large-scale clinical trials regarding PBM for PV, but clinical cases or some clinical approaches have been reported. Therefore, the most therapeutic experience that encouraged the use of PBM to treat PV lesions is probably derived from few case reports that described wound healing after PBM on patients with other types of recalcitrant lesions. Therefore, we recommend that PBM should be used as a coadjutant tool for PV patients in a context of burden resulted from conventional therapies side effects or symptomatic ulcers resistant to healing (Table 18.1).

Table 18.1 Photobiomodulation parameters suggested for treating pemphigus vulgaris[a]

Wavelength (nm)		Red: 660
Power (mW)		100
Radiant energy (J)		2/point
Fluence (J/cm^2)		2
Photonic fluence	(p.J/cm^2)	≈ 3.8
	(Einstein)	≈ 0.8
Exposure time (s/point)		20
Spot location		3–4 points above and around each blister
Treatment days		Every day or alternate days until complete healing[b]

[a]Corticosteroids are the gold standard treatment for PV. PBM should be used for cases where traditional treatments had previously failed, to accelerate healing and pain relief
[b]Clinicians should prioritize pain relief after diagnosis is made and the treatment with corticosteroids is initiated

Treatment

- *Systemic Pharmacological Treatment*
  - Analgesics and corticosteroids
- *Topical Pharmacological Treatment*
  - Anesthetics topical agents
  - Corticosteroids
- *Photobiomodulation*

Further Reading

Amadori F, Bardellini E, Veneri F, Majorana A. Photobiomodulation laser therapy in pemphigus vulgaris oral lesions: a randomized, double-blind, controlled study. Stomatologija. 2022;24(3):80–4.

Dal Prá KJ, de Assis Tristão SDSS, Franco JB, Matias DT, Carrillo CM, de Melo Peres MPS, Ribas PF. Oral management of pemphigus vulgaris in the intensive care unit. Spec Care Dentist. 2020 May;40(3):280–4.

de Carvalho MM, Hidalgo MAR, Scarel-Caminaga RM, Ribeiro Junior NV, Sperandio FF, Pigossi SC, de Carli ML. Photobiomodulation of gingival lesions resulting from autoimmune diseases: systematic review and meta-analysis. Clin Oral Investig. 2022 May;26(5):3949–64.

Minicucci EM, Miot HA, Barraviera SR, Almeida-Lopes L. Low-level laser therapy on the treatment of oral and cutaneous pemphigus vulgaris: case report. Lasers Med Sci. 2012;27:1103–6.

Nili A, Salehi Farid A, Asgari M, Tavakolpour S, Mahmoudi H, Daneshpazhooh M. Current status and prospects for the diagnosis of pemphigus vulgaris. Expert Rev Clin Immunol. 2021 Aug;17(8):819–34.

Yousef M, Mansouri P, Partovikia M, Esmaili M, Younespour S, Hassani L. The effect of low-level laser therapy on pemphigus vulgaris lesions: a pilot study. J Lasers Med Sci. 2017;8:177–80.

Chapter 19
Mucous Membrane Pemphigoid

Mariana Villarroel-Dorrego, Roberto Gerber-Mora, Vinicius Coelho Carrard, and Cristina Saldivia-Siracusa

Disease Definition

Mucous membrane pemphigoid (MMP) is a chronic, autoimmune disease with subepithelial blistering and erosive lesions on the oral mucosa, on other sites of head and neck region and other areas of trauma on human body. Microscopically, the disease is defined by the presence of autoantibodies against the dermal–epidermal junction and predominant involvement of mucous membranes. Diagnosis is made by the clinical presentation and linear deposits of IgG and/or IgA and/or C3 at the dermal–epidermal junction by DIF microscopy of a perilesional biopsy.

MMP usually has a late onset, between the ages of 60 and 80 years. Women appear to be more commonly affected than men. The initial signs and symptoms may be subtle and nonspecific, with irreversible and often debilitating consequences. It is a chronic, progressive condition that most often affects the head and neck region at the oral mucosa (85% of patients), followed by the ocular conjunctiva (65%), nasal mucosa (20–40%), skin (25–30%), pharynx (20%), and larynx (5–15%).

M. Villarroel-Dorrego (✉)
Dental Research Institute, School of Dentistry, Central University of Venezuela, Caracas, Venezuela
e-mail: mariana.villarroel@ucv.ve

R. Gerber-Mora
Oroclínica, Private Practice, San José, Costa Rica

V. C. Carrard
School of Dentistry, Federal University of Rio Grande do Sul, Porto Alegre, RS, Brazil

C. Saldivia-Siracusa
Oral Diagnosis Department, Piracicaba Dental School, University of Campinas, Piracicaba, SP, Brazil

A. R. Santos-Silva et al. (eds.), *Photobiomodulation Therapy in Oral Medicine*,
https://doi.org/10.1007/978-3-031-85048-6_19

The oral cavity and the gingival tissues are the most affected sites. MMP does not have a predictable natural history. Involvement of the oral mucosa typically manifests as erythematous plaques and erosions that are covered by pseudomembrane, most located on the gingiva and palate and less frequently on the lips, tongue, and buccal mucosa. Gingival lesions are often described as desquamative gingivitis and also found in lichen planus and pemphigus vulgaris.

A multidisciplinary approach involving dermatologists, oral medicine specialists, and other healthcare professionals is often necessary to address the complex and diverse manifestations of MMP and improve the quality of life for affected individuals.

Diagnosis

- Clinical evaluation
- Perilesional biopsy
- Direct immunofluorescence microscopy

Treatment

Topical and systemic corticosteroids have been indicated as the most effective method for treatment of oral lesions resulting from autoimmune disorders. MMP does not diverge from this scenario. However, MMP patients may respond differently to a given therapy, and the adverse effects of corticosteroids require new alternatives of treatment. As discussed throughout this book, the use of systemic steroids presents an increased risk of adverse effects. Photobiomodulation (PBM) has been suggested to treat oral lesions of autoimmune etiologies (such as MMP). In this context, PBM has been proposed in case reports in the literature for pain relief and wound healing, when associated with systemic and topical immunosuppressive therapies.

However, the pooled results of literature comparing the use of PBM to corticosteroids regarding pain management of autoimmune oral lesions suggest that there is no significant difference between tested groups. Although the use of PBM alone or in conjunction with corticosteroids seems promising, a recent meta-analysis also demonstrated that laser parameters used in different studies showed great variation respecting wavelengths, ranging from 308 to 10,600 nm, and power output from 0.007 to 3W, making it difficult to establish a reliable protocol. In summary, PBM may be as effective as topical corticosteroids for symptoms relief. Therefore, the authors of the present chapter recommend PBM as an option for patients with restrictions on the use of corticosteroids since there are few studies available to ensure the role of PBM for oral lesions derived from autoimmune disorders (Table 19.1).

Table 19.1 Photobiomodulation parameters suggested for treating Mucous membrane pemphigoid[a]

Wavelength (nm)		Red: 660	NIR: 810–970
Power (mW)		30–100	100–300
Radiant energy (J)		2/point	3/point
Fluence (J/cm²)		1	3
Photonic fluence	(p.J/cm²)	≈ 1.9	≈ 3.9–4.5
	(Einstein)	≈ 0.4	≈ 0.8–1
Exposure time (s/point)		10	
Spot location		Mucosal lesions and the perilesional tissue	
Treatment days		Every day or alternate days until complete healing[b]	

MMP mucous membrane pemphigoid
[a]Corticosteroids are the gold standard treatment for MMP. Studies herein presented suggest that PBM should be used for cases where traditional treatments had previously failed, to accelerate healing and pain relief
[b]Clinicians should prioritize pain relief after diagnosis is made and the treatment with corticosteroids is initiated

Treatment

- *Systemic Pharmacological Treatment*
  - Analgesics
    It is recommended to discuss with the patient's physician the prescription of opioids to ensure the most suitable analgesic protocol. Physicians usually consider all steps of pain management scale when prescribing analgesics.
  - Systemic corticosteroids
- *Topical Pharmacological Treatment*
  - Corticosteroids
  - Anesthetics topical agents
- *Photobiomodulation*

Further Reading

Cafaro A, Broccoletti R, Arduino PG. Low-level laser therapy for oral mucous membrane pemphigoid. Lasers Med Sci. 2012;27:1247–50.

de Carvalho MM, Hidalgo MAR, Scarel-Caminaga RM, Ribeiro Junior NV, Sperandio FF, Pigossi SC, de Carli ML. Photobiomodulation of gingival lesions resulting from autoimmune diseases: systematic review and meta-analysis. Clin Oral Investig. 2022 May;26(5):3949–64.

Oliveira PC, Reis Junior JA, Lacerda JA, Silveira NT, Santos JM, Vitale MC, Pinheiro AL. Laser light may improve the symptoms of oral lesions of cicatricial pemphigoid: a case report. Photomed Laser Surg. 2009;27:825–8.

Taylor J, McMillan R, Shephard M, Setterfield J, Ahmed R, Carrozzo M, Grando S, Mignogna M, Kuten-Shorrer M, Musbah T, Elia A, McGowan R, Kerr AR, Greenberg MS, Hodgson T, Sirois D. World workshop on oral medicine VI: a systematic review of the treatment of mucous membrane pemphigoid. Oral Surg Oral Med Oral Pathol Oral Radiol. 2015 Aug;120(2):161–71.e20.

Yilmaz HG, Kusakci-Seker B, Bayindir H, Tözüm TF. Low-level laser therapy in the treatment of mucous membrane pemphigoid: a promising procedure. J Periodontol. 2010 Aug;81(8):1226–30.

Chapter 20
Geographic Tongue

Lara Eunice Cândido Soares, Danielle Martins Startari, Ana Carolina Prado Ribeiro, and Juliana Lucena Schussel

Disease Definition

Geographic tongue (GT), also known as benign migratory glossitis, is characterized as an inflammatory disorder with an unknown etiology. The clinical presentation of geographic tongue can be described as red and circular areas with white borders, mainly located in the dorsum and border of the tongue, and assembles to a map, which is a result of filiform papillae atrophy. Interestingly, the size and shape of lesions constantly change.

Although the precise etiology of GT remains unclear, it has been associated with several conditions, such as:

- Emotional stress
- Vitamin deficiency
- Genetic predisposition
- Immune disorders, among others

L. E. C. Soares
Private Practice, Teresina, PI, Brazil

D. M. Startari
Private Practice, Campo Grande, MS, Brazil

Oral Diagnosis Department, Piracicaba Dental School, University of Campinas, Piracicaba, SP, Brazil

A. C. P. Ribeiro
Dental Oncology Service, São Paulo State Cancer Institute, University of São Paulo Medical School, São Paulo, SP, Brazil

J. L. Schussel (✉)
Department of Stomatology, Federal University of Paraná, Curitiba, PR, Brazil

A. R. Santos-Silva et al. (eds.), *Photobiomodulation Therapy in Oral Medicine*,
https://doi.org/10.1007/978-3-031-85048-6_20

GT is estimated to have a prevalence of ≈2–3%, with no gender predisposition. This condition is typically asymptomatic, but some individuals may experience discomfort or sensitivity with periods of exacerbation and remission. The occurrence of concurrent lingual fissures is commonly observed and may impact the severity of associated symptoms. GT does not have a cure, and it usually does not require treatment, but interventions may be necessary when lesions are symptomatic (burning sensation and taste diminution).

Diagnosis

- Clinical evaluation

Treatment

As mentioned above, GT has no cure. However, clinicians may treat its symptoms when patients report to be necessary. There is no gold standard protocol for treating GT. Therefore, professionals may need to have a comprehensive overview of the patient's symptoms and establish a personalized treatment plan. The most common therapeutic regimens include the use of steroids or immunosuppressive topical therapies.

Recent findings from a randomized clinical trial have demonstrated that photobiomodulation (PBM) effectively alleviated the discomfort associated with GT. Differently to what is commonly attributed to PBM, this approach will not induce accelerated healing but only in symptoms relief. However, PBM may be a promising alternative to medication-based treatments (Table 20.1) because it may reduce side effects of non-curable diseases–such as GT–that require long-term drug therapy.

Table 20.1 Photobiomodulation parameters suggested for treating geographic tongue

Wavelength (nm)		Red: 660
Power (mW)		25
Radiant energy (J)		3/point
Fluence (J/cm^2)		3
Photonic fluence	(p.J/cm^2)	≈ 5.7
	(Einstein)	≈ 1.2
Exposure time (s/point)		120
Spot location		All affected area
Treatment days		Every day until complete resolution of symptoms

Treatment

- *Systemic Pharmacological Treatment*
  - Analgesics
- *Topical Pharmacological Treatment*
  - Corticosteroids
- *Photobiomodulation*

Further Reading

de Campos WG, Esteves CV, Fernandes LG, Domaneschi C, Júnior CAL. Treatment of symptomatic benign migratory glossitis: a systematic review. Clin Oral Investig. 2018 Sep;22(7):2487–93.
Lucchese A, Di Stasio D, De Stefano S, Nardone M, Carinci F. Beyond the gut: a systematic review of oral manifestations in celiac disease. J Clin Med. 2023 Jun 6;12(12):3874.
Pereira RDPL, de Oliveira JMD, Pauletto P, Munhoz EA, Silva Guerra EN, Massignan C, De Luca Canto G. Worldwide prevalence of geographic tongue in adults: a systematic review and meta-analysis. Oral Dis. 2023 Nov;29(8):3091–100.
Saad I. Photobiomodulation effect of low-level laser therapy as a palliative treatment of symptomatic geographic tongue (a double-blinded randomized clinical trial). J Contemp Dent Pract. 2020;21:453–7.
Sarruf MBJM, Quinelato V, Sarruf GJM, Oliveira HE, Calasans-Maia JA, Quinelato H, Aguiar T, Casado PL, Cavalcante LMA. Stress as worsening of the signs and symptoms of the geographic tongue during the COVID-19 pandemic: a pilot study. BMC Oral Health. 2022 Dec 3;22(1):565.

Chapter 21
Burning Mouth Syndrome

Thaís Cristina Esteves-Pereira, Ana Gabriela Costa Normando, Marcio Ajudarte Lopes, and Alan Roger Santos-Silva

Disease Definition

Burning mouth syndrome (BMS), previous known as glossodynia, is characterized by a burning sensation and discomfort that affects the oral mucosa without local or systemic cause. The International Headache Society (IHS) currently defines BMS as an intraoral burning or dysesthetic sensation that occurs daily for >2 h for >3 months, unaccompanied by somatosensory changes and without evident causative lesions on clinical examination and investigation. Global prevalence estimates that BMS affects 1.73% of general population, with higher prevalence for those over 50 years. A predilection for women is seen, mainly those with 50–60 decades of life, with incidence of almost 20% for postmenopausal population.

According to the updated classification of orofacial pain by the International Classification of Orofacial Pain (ICOP), the BMS diagnostic criteria includes (A) oral pain fulfilling the criteria B and C, (B) recurring daily for >2 h per day for >3 months, (C) pain has both of the following characteristics: (C1) burning quality and (C2) felt superficially in the oral mucosa, (D) oral mucosa is of normal appearance and local or systemic causes have been excluded, and (E) not better accounted by another ICOP or International Classification of Headache Disorders—third version (ICHD-3) diagnosis.

The IHS has classified primary BMS as a neuropathy of idiopathic nature, with peripheral and central components, and no longer is considered a psychogenic pain. Primary or idiopathic BMS is classified into two main subtypes: peripheral or central. The central subtype usually does not respond to local treatments and is often associated with a psychiatric comorbidity (most commonly depression or anxiety), whereas the peripheral subtype reacts to topical treatments modalities. If the

T. C. Esteves-Pereira (✉) · A. G. C. Normando · M. A. Lopes · A. R. Santos-Silva
Oral Diagnosis Department, Piracicaba Dental School, University of Campinas, Piracicaba, SP, Brazil

A. R. Santos-Silva et al. (eds.), *Photobiomodulation Therapy in Oral Medicine*,
https://doi.org/10.1007/978-3-031-85048-6_21

burning sensation can be explained by a local (candidiasis, lichen planus, and hyposalivation) or systemic disorder (medication induced, anemia, deficiencies of vitamin B12 or folic acid, Sjögren's syndrome, and diabetes), it is classified as secondary BMS.

Xerostomia is the most frequent symptom in BMS besides burning and may be attributed to stress, anxiety, and somatization. Sialorrhea, although uncommon, has been reported in BMS patients. Furthermore, taste alterations (biter or metallic) and changes in patient's daily diet may be reported as spice and hot food often results in symptoms worsening. Besides a burning and painful sensations, xerostomia and dysgeusia may occur mostly affecting the anterior two-thirds of the tongue, followed by the gingiva, palate, and labial mucosa. The literature shows that depression and anxiety are associated with BMS, despite no direct cause-and-effect relationship has been established.

Although the exact pathogenesis of BMS remains unclear, some studies have suggested a multifactorial nature, in which local (e.g., lower levels of proteoglycans, greater amount of collagen fibers, fewer intraepithelial nerve fibers, and compromised local thermal neurofunction) and physiological factors (stress, anxiety, depression, and sleep disorders) are assumed as potential etiological causes. Besides, studies have suggested a possible dysfunction at several levels of the neuronal axis, such as whiter matter and temporal lobe alterations.

Health-related and oral health-related quality of life in BMS patients is poor, highlighting the impact of the disease in physical and psychosocial state of patients. Managing BMS can be frustrating for clinicians due to its challenging symptoms, and it can often be a burden for patients since it is an incurable condition. It is important to note that BMS severely affects patients' well-being.

Diagnosis

- History and clinical evaluation.
  The patient's medical history, list of medications, and the establishment of symptoms characteristics (onset, site, time course, exacerbating/relieving factors, and severity) provide valuable insights for the diagnostic process, particularly considering the fulfillment of the diagnostic criteria proposed by the ICOP.
- Hematologic exam evaluation.
  - Nutritional deficiencies (e.g., iron, zinc, folic acid, and vitamin B complex).
  - Autoimmune disorders and hormonal imbalances.
  - Viral culture and fungal culture (oral infections).
- Lingual nerve block.

The lingual nerve block is a helpful tool for diagnostic purposes, proposed by Grémeau-Richard et al. (2010). This technique was proposed to assist clinicians in differentiating between central and peripheral idiopathic BMS. When the lingual nerve is blocked and the burning pain is completely relieved, the patient is considered to have peripheral BMS. In contrast, in patients with central BMS, the sensation persists or even intensifies following the nerve block.

Treatment

It is not surprising that no specific therapy for BMS is available considering what was discussed above. Thus, no significant advances have been reported in recent studies, and its management is centered on symptoms relief, as a definitive cure seems to be a distant reality. Among the medications used for BMS management, antidepressants, antipsychotics, antiepileptics, and analgesics have been described as the category of drugs that has the most effective results. In addition to these drugs, dietary chances by means of vitamin and mineral supplementations and hormonal replacement have been described as potential therapeutic approaches, but no hard conclusion could be drawn.

Photobiomodulation (PBM) has been recommended to treat BMS as several studies evaluated its efficacy. The rationale for using PBM in individuals with BMS is based on its physiologicals mechanisms. PBM may increase the production of serotonin and the release of β-endorphins, inhibit the depolarization of C-fibers, reduce bradykinin secretion, and promote ATP synthesis. This biological process is what enables the analgesic effect of low-level laser appliances. The currently available evidence suggests that the red laser is preferred for pain relief, but it does not permit a definitive conclusion regarding the superiority of red laser over infrared laser. Consequently, it is not possible to provide a singular standard of application, as displayed in Table 21.1. Novel randomized controlled clinical trials are currently

Table 21.1 Photobiomodulation parameters suggested for treating burning mouth syndrome

Wavelength (nm)		Red: 660	NIR: 810
Power (mW)		100	100–200
Radiant energy (J)		2	3–6
Fluence (J/cm²)		1.5	2
Photonic fluence	(p.J/cm²)	≈ 2.8	≈ 3
	(Einstein)	≈ 0.6	≈ 0.6
Exposure time (s/point)		15	
Spot location		3 points at tip of the tongue, 4 points at lateral tongue, 10 points at dorsal tongue, 8 points at buccal mucosa, 5 points at labial mucosa, 8 points at hard palate, 3 points at soft palate, 3 points/sextant at gingiva, or alveolar mucosa	
Treatment days		1–5 sessions weekly for 4–10 weeks	

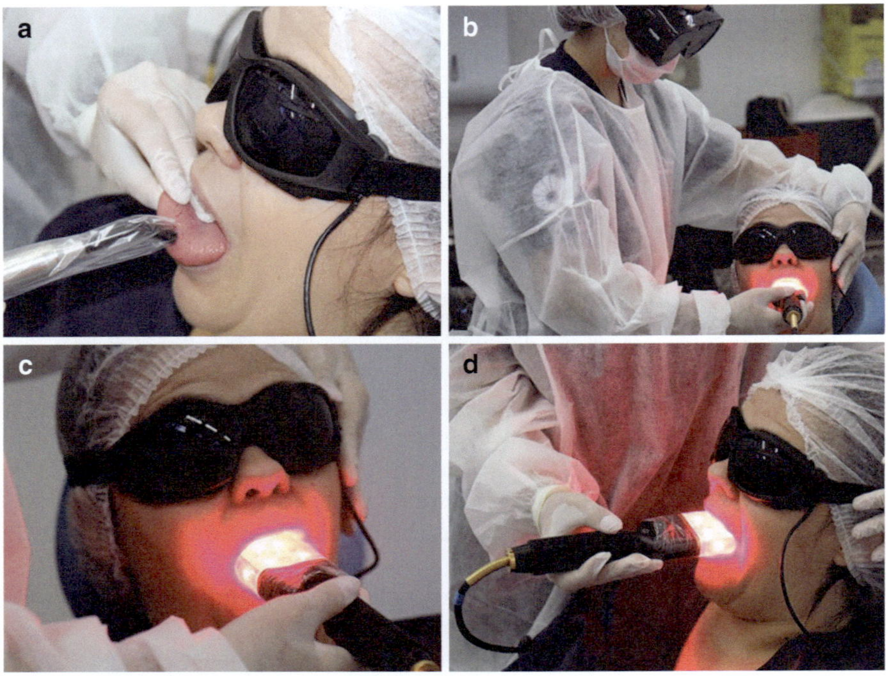

Fig. 21.1 Photobiomodulation therapy for burning mouth syndrome (BMS). (**a**) NIR laser (810 nm) applied to dorsal tongue. (**b–d**). LED Lollipop cluster (660 e 850 nm). (THOR Photomedicine Ltd., Amersham, UK)

underway to address the optimal wavelength and photonic fluence for BMS (Fig. 21.1).

Treatment

- *Systemic Pharmacological Treatment.*
  - Benzodiazepines (clonazepam).
  - Tricyclic antidepressants (amitriptyline and nortriptyline).
  - Anticonvulsants (gabapentin and pregabalin).
  - Alpha-lipoic acid.
- *Topical Pharmacological Treatment.*
  - Capsaicin (mouthwash).
  - Clonazepam (solution and disintegrated table).
- *Photobiomodulation.*

Further Reading

Al-Maweri SA, Javed F, Kalakonda B, AlAizari NA, Al-Soneidar W, Al-Akwa A. Efficacy of low-level laser therapy in the treatment of burning mouth syndrome: a systematic review. Photodiagn Photodyn Ther. 2017;17:188–93.

Ariyawardana A, Chmieliauskaite M, Farag AM, Albuquerque R, Forssell H, Nasri-Heir C, Klasser GD, Sardella A, Mignogna MD, Ingram M, Carlson CR, Miller CS. World Workshop on Oral Medicine VII: Burning mouth syndrome: a systematic review of disease definitions and diagnostic criteria utilized in randomized clinical trials. Oral Dis. 2019 Jun;25(Suppl 1):141–56.

Calderipe CB, Kirschnick LB, Esteves-Pereira TC, Dos Santos ES, Vasconcelos ACU, Lopes MA, Treister NS, Santos-Silva AR. Local anesthesia nerve block for managing burning mouth syndrome: a scoping review. Oral Surg Oral Med Oral Pathol Oral Radiol. 2024 Jul 22;S2212-4403(24):00394–8.

Canfora F, Calabria E, Spagnuolo G, Coppola N, Armogida NG, Mazzaccara C, Solari D, D'Aniello L, Aria M, Pecoraro G, Mignogna MD, Leuci S, Adamo D. Salivary complaints in burning mouth syndrome: a cross sectional study on 500 patients. J Clin Med. 2023 Aug 26;12(17):5561.

de Lima-Souza RA, Pérez-de-Oliveira ME, Normando AGC, Louredo BVR, Mariano FV, Farag AM, Santos-Silva AR. Clinical and epidemiological profile of burning mouth syndrome patients following the International Headache Society classification: a systematic review and meta-analysis. Oral Surg Oral Med Oral Pathol Oral Radiol. 2024 Feb;137(2):119–35.

de Pedro M, López-Pintor RM, Casañas E, Hernández G. Effects of photobiomodulation with low-level laser therapy in burning mouth syndrome: a randomized clinical trial. Oral Dis. 2020;26:1764–76.

Farag AM, Kuten-Shorrer M, Natto Z, Ariyawardana A, Mejia LM, Albuquerque R, Carey B, Chmieliauskaite M, Miller CS, Ingram M, Nasri-Heir C, Sardella A, Carlson CR, Klasser GD. WWOM VII: Effectiveness of systemic pharmacotherapeutic interventions in the management of BMS: a systematic review and meta-analysis. Oral Dis. 2023 Mar;29(2):343–68.

Farag AM, Carey B, Albuquerque R. Oral dysaesthesia: a special focus on aetiopathogenesis, clinical diagnostics and treatment modalities. Br Dent J. 2024 Feb;236(4):275–8.

Gonçalves S, Carey B, Farag AM, Kuten-Shorrer M, Natto ZS, Ariyawardana A, Mejia LM, Chmieliauskaite M, Miller CS, Ingram M, Nasri-Heir C, Sardella A, Carlson CR, Klasser GD, O'Neill F, Albuquerque R. WWOM VII: effectiveness of topical interventions in the management of burning mouth syndrome: a systematic review. Oral Dis. 2023 Nov;29(8):3016–33.

Grémeau-Richard C, Dubray C, Aublet-Cuvelier B, Ughetto S, Woda A. Effect of lingual nerve block on burning mouth syndrome (stomatodynia): a randomized crossover trial. Pain. 2010 Apr;149(1):27–32.

Headache Classification Committee of the International Headache Society (IHS). The International Classification of Headache Disorders, 3rd edition (beta version). Cephalalgia. 2013 Jul;33(9):629–808.

Headache Classification Committee of the International Headache Society (IHS). The international classification of headache disorders, 3rd edition. Cephalalgia. 2018 Jan;38(1):1–211.

International Classification of Orofacial Pain, 1st edition (ICOP). Cephalalgia 2020;40(2):129–221.

Marotta BM, Sugaya NN, Hanna R, Gallo CB. Efficacy of 660 nm Photobiomodulation in burning mouth syndrome management: a single-blind quasi-experimental controlled clinical trial. Photobiomodul Photomed Laser Surg. 2024 Mar;42(3):225–9.

McMillan R, Forssell H, Buchanan JA, Glenny AM, Weldon JC, Zakrzewska JM. Interventions for treating burning mouth syndrome. Cochrane Database Syst Rev. 2016 Nov 18;11(11):CD002779.

Pereira JV, Normando AGC, Rodrigues-Fernandes CI, Rivera C, Santos-Silva AR, Lopes MA. The impact on quality of life in patients with burning mouth syndrome: a systematic review and meta-analysis. Oral Surg Oral Med Oral Pathol Oral Radiol. 2021;131:186–94.

Santos-Silva AR, Villa A. The multidimensional impact of burning mouth syndrome on patients and their families. Oral Dis. 2024 Nov;30(8):4819–20.

Spanemberg JC, Segura-Egea JJ, Rodríguez-de Rivera-Campillo E, Jané-Salas E, Salum FG, López-López J. Low-level laser therapy in patients with burning mouth syndrome: a double-blind, randomized, controlled clinical trial. J Clin Exp Dent. 2019;11:e162–9.

Wu S, Zhang W, Yan J, Noma N, Young A, Yan Z. Worldwide prevalence estimates of burning mouth syndrome: a systematic review and meta-analysis. Oral Dis. 2022 Sep;28(6):1431–40.

Chapter 22
Neuropathic Pain

Sven Eric Niklander, Markéta Janovská, and Arwa Mohammad Farag

Disease Definition

The International Association for the Study of Pain (IASP) defines neuropathic pain (NP) as "pain caused by a lesion or disease of the somatosensory system", replacing the definition in the Classification of Chronic Pain published by IASP, 1994. NP may occur particularly due to peripheral nerve lesion (amputation), infection (post herpetic neuralgia), or exposure to neurotoxins. Other possible causes of NP are chemotherapy, radiation, nerve compression (accidents, surgeries, and tumor infiltration), infarction (ischemia respectively), inflammation, metabolic disorders (diabetic neuralgia) or neurodegenerative conditions, vitamin deficiencies or can also be idiopathic.

NP in orofacial region is traditionally divided into episodic (trigeminal neuralgia) and continuous (post-traumatic trigeminal neuropathic pain and postherpetic neuralgia). Main characteristics of NP include pain quality, which is mostly burning, tingling, and resembling of electric shock or might be itching or pricking. NP can be accompanied by somatosensory impairments such as hypoesthesia (reduced

S. E. Niklander (✉)
Department of Oral Pathology and Surgery, School of Dentistry, Universidad Andres Bello, Viña del Mar, Chile
e-mail: sven.niklander@unab.cl

M. Janovská
Department of Oral Medicine, Institute of Dental Medicine, First Faculty of Medicine and General University Hospital, Charles University, Prague, Czech Republic

A. M. Farag
Department of Oral Diagnostic Sciences, King Abdulaziz University Faculty of Dentistry, Jeddah, Saudi Arabia

Department of Diagnostic Sciences, School of Dental Medicine, Tufts University, Boston, MA, USA

A. R. Santos-Silva et al. (eds.), *Photobiomodulation Therapy in Oral Medicine*,
https://doi.org/10.1007/978-3-031-85048-6_22

sensitivity to stimulation), allodynia (pain arising from stimulus that would not cause pain in standard situation), paresthesia (abnormal pain sensation), or hyperalgesia (increased pain following stimulus that normally causes pain). Of note, stimulation of nociceptor might not be essential. NP typically follows the course of the affected nerve and persists long-term even after tissue damage has resolved.

The physiopathology and its biological mechanisms remain enigmatic, but according to the International Classification of Orofacial Pain 2020 (ICOP-2020), NP can be classified as central or peripheral, according to the location of the nervous lesion. Peripheral mechanisms are purported to nerve inflammatory response to trigeminal nerve injury and peripheral neuronal hyperexcitability when noninjured axons are activated. Central sensitization is thought to be related to hyperresponsiveness of central neurons when spinal and supraspinal nociceptive pathways are abundantly or frequently stimulated and become more sensitive to ensuing stimuli.

Diagnosis

- Clinical evaluation
- Patient's thorough history (including any history of trauma to orofacial region) with detailed interpretation of symptoms (onset, character, and distribution of pain) and any precipitating factors and associated symptoms such as sensory disturbances
- Quantitative sensory testing (spatula test, cotton swab test, or pinprick test) measuring sensory threshold for pain
- Magnetic resonance imaging and magnetic resonance angiography

Treatment

For episodic NP (e.g., trigeminal neuralgia), antiepileptics (phenytoin, pregabalin, gabapentin, and lamotrigine), anticonvulsants (carbamazepine and oxcarbazepine), or baclofen can be treatment of choice. Continuous NP might be managed with low dose of tricyclic antidepressants (e.g., amitriptyline), in some cases with topicals (e.g., capsaicin), antiepileptics (pregabalin or gabapentin), serotonin–norepinephrine reuptake inhibitor (duloxetine), or opioids. Pain control medications are the most used techniques to treat NP symptoms. However, they have shown only 30% effectiveness, in only 50% of the patient population, while their prolonged intake is tied to several adverse effects. Therefore, investigators have been seeking alternative therapeutic modalities, such as anesthetics, neurosensory barriers, neurosurgical procedures, and psychotherapy (cognitive behavioral therapy).

Table 22.1 Photobiomodulation parameters suggested for treating neuropathic pain

Wavelength (nm)		NIR: 780–905
Power (mW)		70
Radiant energy (J)		1–10/point
Fluence (J/cm^2)		2.1
Photonic fluence	(p.J/cm^2)	≈ 2.9–3.3
	(Einstein)	≈ 0.6–0.7
Exposure time (s/point)		30
Spot location		Trigger points or the area indicated by the patient
Treatment days		Daily for 2 weeks

Photobiomodulation (PBM) has emerged as a prominent focus in investigations related to tissue regeneration and pain reduction. While certain clinical trials have demonstrated positive outcomes with PBM for NP, it is noteworthy that laser parameters have exhibited significant variability. Establishing a singular configuration has proven challenging; however, there appears to be a discernible "therapeutic window" associated with satisfactory results. Therefore, Table 22.1 will display the smallest window possible disregarding the devices with high energy density parameters, considering the possibility that the majority of dentists will work with without high energy density laser apparatus.

Treatment

- *Systemic Pharmacological Treatment*
  - Analgesics
  - Antiepileptics (phenytoin, pregabalin, gabapentin, and lamotrigine)
  - Anticonvulsants (carbamazepine and oxcarbazepine)
  - Baclofen
  - Tricyclic antidepressants (amitriptyline)
  - Serotonin–norepinephrine reuptake inhibitors (duloxetine)
  - Opioids
- *Topical Pharmacological Treatment*
  - Anesthetics topical agents
  - Capsaicin
- *Surgical treatment*
  - Neurosurgical procedures
- *Miscellaneous*
  - Psychotherapy
  - Physiotherapy
- *Photobiomodulation*

Further Reading

Attal N, Cruccu G, Baron R, Haanpää M, Hansson P, Jensen TS, Nurmikko T. EFNS guidelines on the pharmacological treatment of neuropathic pain: 2010 revision. Eur J Neurol. 2010 Sep;17(9):1113–e88.

Backonja M, Woolf CJ. Future directions in neuropathic pain therapy: closing the translational loop. Oncologist. 2010;15(Suppl 2):24–9.

de Andrade AL, Bossini PS, Parizotto NA. Use of low-level laser therapy to control neuropathic pain: a systematic review. J Photochem Photobiol B. 2016;164:36–42.

de Pedro M, López-Pintor RM, de la Hoz-Aizpurua JL, Casañas E, Hernández G. Efficacy of low-level laser therapy for the therapeutic management of neuropathic orofacial pain: a systematic review. J Oral Facial Pain Headache. 2020;34:13–30.

International Classification of Orofacial Pain, 1st edition (ICOP). Cephalalgia 2020;40(2):129–221.

Meacham K, Shepherd A, Mohapatra DP, Haroutounian S. Neuropathic pain: central vs. peripheral mechanisms. Curr Pain Headache Rep. 2017;21(6):28.

Scholz J, Finnerup NB, Attal N, Aziz Q, Baron R, Bennett MI, Benoliel R, Cohen M, Cruccu G, Davis KD, Evers S, First M, Giamberardino MA, Hansson P, Kaasa S, Korwisi B, Kosek E, Lavand'homme P, Nicholas M, Nurmikko T, Perrot S, Raja SN, Rice ASC, Rowbotham MC, Schug S, Simpson DM, Smith BH, Svensson P, Vlaeyen JWS, Wang SJ, Barke A, Rief W, Treede RD, Classification Committee of the Neuropathic Pain Special Interest Group (NeuPSIG). The IASP classification of chronic pain for ICD-11: chronic neuropathic pain. Pain. 2019;160(1):53–9.

Shinoda M, Imamura Y, Hayashi Y, Noma N, Okada-Ogawa A, Hitomi S, Iwata K. Orofacial neuropathic pain-basic research and their clinical relevancies. Front Mol Neurosci. 2021;14:691396.

Chapter 23
Trigeminal Neuralgia

Manoela Carrera, Marco Antônio Trevizani Martins, and Manoela Domingues Martins

Disease Definition

Trigeminal neuralgia (TN) is one of the most painful conditions of the head and neck region. Its occurrence is more often described in female patients at 50 years of age or elderly, as well. Although rare, TN may also affect younger adults (< 40 years old) or even children. In general, it is estimated that TN affects 1:15,000–25,000 patients. However, TN is frequently misdiagnosis, and its prevalence data may be even higher. TN is described as a unilateral sharp pain like an electric shock or a perforation that starts suddenly or triggered by an ordinary action (e.g., washing, shaving, talking, brushing teeth, or even a gentle contact to mucosa or skin), at a specific area named as "trigger points". Sometimes, with severe pain, facial muscle spasms can be seen. Hence, TN is also known as "tic douloureux".

Most common sites include perinasal and oral skin, lips, cheeks, eyebrows and tongue. There are some patients who have been described to the authors of the present chapter that the smooth touch of a piece of cotton at the trigger point may initiate the pain episodes.

M. Carrera (✉)
Faculty of Dentistry, Federal University of Bahia, Salvador, BA, Brazil

State University of Bahia, Salvador, BA, Brazil

M. A. T. Martins
Department of Oral Medicine, Porto Alegre Clinics Hospital, Porto Alegre, RS, Brazil

Department of Oral Pathology, School of Dentistry, Federal University of Rio Grande do Sul, Porto Alegre, RS, Brazil

M. D. Martins
Department of Oral Pathology, School of Dentistry, Federal University of Rio Grande do Sul, Porto Alegre, RS, Brazil

A. R. Santos-Silva et al. (eds.), *Photobiomodulation Therapy in Oral Medicine*,
https://doi.org/10.1007/978-3-031-85048-6_23

Pain can last seconds, but the patient's quality of life is dramatically affected–as it is characteristic of this condition–in which some suicidal desire may be manifested by some individuals to end their suffering. It can be experienced from a single attack during the day to more than one attack per minute. Regarding symptomatology, TN can be classified into type 1, in which there is a presence of paroxysmal pain alone, or type 2, characterized by paroxysmal pain along with constant pain in the background. The most involved branches are maxillary or mandibular division.

The International Headache Society (IHS) classifies TN into three categories based on the pain's origin: Classic TN includes TN related to vascular compression, secondary TN includes TN due to a tumor along the trigeminal nerve or TN due to an underlying disease like multiple sclerosis, and idiopathic TN is defined as TN with an unknown cause.

Although image exams may help by excluding some other hypotheses, the clinical evaluation and patient interview are sufficient to establish the diagnosis. However, theories of the TN pathogenicity are divided into peripheral and central. The first (peripheral) theory describes changes in peripheral axon and myelin, resulting to altered chemical and physical stimuli. The central pathogenicity theory is based on a similarity between TN and focal epilepsy, in which there is pressure on nerve branches or ganglia. Interestingly, some researchers believe both central and peripheral mechanisms may act simultaneously.

Diagnosis

- Clinical evaluation

  Differential diagnosis might include postherpetic neuralgia and temporomandibular dysfunction.

- Brain magnetic resonance imaging

Treatment

To date, the first line of treatment includes anti-inflammatories, powerful analgesics, and anticonvulsant drugs. Tolerance may be developed, and the need for extra dosage increases, leading to more side effects. Therefore, nearly 50% of TN patients experience incomplete control of pain or drug-related side effects. In this context, surgical procedures, such as trigeminal root section, sectioning of the trigeminal tract in the lower medulla, and microvascular decompression, have been proposed. Despite drug and surgical therapies promote a certain level of symptom relief, there are significant risks and adverse effects that create a demand for new treatments.

Table 23.1 Photobiomodulation parameters suggested for treating trigeminal neuralgia

Wavelength (nm)		NIR: 810–830
Power (mW)		200
Radiant energy (J)		5/point
Fluence (J/cm^2)		5
Photonic fluence	(p.J/cm^2)	≈ 7.5
	(Einstein)	≈ 1.6
Exposure time (s/point)		25
Spot location		Trigger points or the path of pain indicated by the patient
Treatment days		1–2 sessions/week for 8 weeks

PBM therapy has emerged as an interesting treatment option in patients with neuralgias (e.g., postherpetic and trigeminal) and neurodegenerative diseases. Therefore, these therapeutic experiences encouraged the suggestion that PBM may induce pain relief without any side effects for TN. It may also be an interesting adjuvant tool for those patients tolerant to drug therapies. Most of the studies available in literature evaluated the NIR range of light, probably because this wavelength induces more neuroprotection effects (such as neurogenesis, new pathways, and stimulation of neural cells). Table 23.1 displays the suggested PBM parameters for TN.

Treatment

- *Systemic Pharmacological Treatment*
  - Analgesics
  - Carbamazepine
  - Phenytoin baclofen
  - Gabapentin
  - Oxcarbazepine
  - Lamotrigine
- *Topical Pharmacological Treatment*
  - Glycerol injections
- *Miscellaneous*
  - Percutaneous radiofrequency thermocoagulation
- *Botulinum Toxin Injection*
- *Photobiomodulation*

Further Reading

de Pedro M, López-Pintor RM, de la Hoz-Aizpurua JL, Casañas E, Hernández G. Efficacy of low-level laser therapy for the therapeutic management of neuropathic orofacial pain: a systematic review. J Oral Facial Pain Headache. 2020;34:13–30.

Ebrahimi H, Najafi S, Khayamzadeh M, Zahedi A, Mahdavi A. Therapeutic and analgesic efficacy of laser in conjunction with pharmaceutical therapy for trigeminal neuralgia. J Lasers Med Sci. 2018;9:63–8.

Falaki F, Nejat AH, Dalirsani Z. The Effect of low-level laser therapy on trigeminal neuralgia: a review of literature. J Dent Res Dent Clin Dent Prospects. 2014;8:1–5.

Headache Classification Committee of the International Headache Society (IHS). The International Classification of Headache Disorders, 3rd edition. Cephalalgia. 2018 Jan;38(1):1–211.

Ibarra AMC, Biasotto-Gonzalez DA, Kohatsu EYI, de Oliveira SSI, Bussadori SK, Tanganeli JPC. Photobiomodulation on trigeminal neuralgia: systematic review. Lasers Med Sci. 2021 Jun;36(4):715–22.

Shankar Kikkeri N, Nagalli S. Trigeminal neuralgia. 2024 Mar 3. StatPearls [Internet]. Treasure Island (FL): StatPearls; 2024 Jan.

Yadav YR, Nishtha Y, Sonjjay P, Vijay P, Shailendra R, Yatin K. Trigeminal Neuralgia. Asian J Neurosurg. 2017 Oct–Dec;12(4):585–97.

Chapter 24
Facial Palsy

Arwa Mohammad Farag, Beatriz Nascimento Figueiredo Lebre Martins, and César Augusto Migliorati

Disease Definition

Facial palsy (FP) is an acute neuromotor disorder affecting the function of the seventh cranial nerve (i.e., facial nerve) predominantly leading to hemifacial paralysis. Approximately 70% of FP cases are idiopathic, known as Bell's palsy. However, viral infections, mainly herpes simplex virus, are believed to be the most common etiologic factor, resulting in nerve inflammation, edema, demyelination, and ischemia. On the other hand, trauma, bony canal stenosis, and iatrogenic chemical/radiation/mechanical injuries to the facial nerve were reported to constitute 20% of the pathoetiologic factors, leaving 10% of the cases to be attributed to either neoplasms or other infections (i.e., bacterial otitis media or herpes zoster induced Ramsay Hunt syndrome). Hyperglycemia, uncontrolled hypertension, preeclampsia, and migraine are among the theorized risk factors that may contribute to the pathophysiology of the disease.

A. M. Farag (✉)
Department of Oral Diagnostic Sciences, King Abdulaziz University Faculty of Dentistry, Jeddah, Saudi Arabia

Department of Diagnostic Sciences, School of Dental Medicine, Tufts University, Boston, MA, USA
e-mail: Arwa.Farag@tufts.edu

B. N. F. L. Martins
Oral Diagnosis Department, Piracicaba Dental School, University of Campinas, Piracicaba, SP, Brazil

C. A. Migliorati
Department of Oral and Maxillofacial Diagnostic Sciences, College of Dentistry, University of Florida, Gainesville, FL, USA

A. R. Santos-Silva et al. (eds.), *Photobiomodulation Therapy in Oral Medicine*,
https://doi.org/10.1007/978-3-031-85048-6_24

The incidence of FP ranges between 15 and 35 cases per 100,000 with an equal gender and a wide age range distribution (i.e., 50–75% of reported cases were between 15 and 50 years old).

The condition is manifested as an acute unilateral progression of facial muscle paralysis that peaks within 48–72 h. Regular oral functions, including eating, drinking, speaking, and other activities, such as eye blinking and eyebrow raising, are affected leading to a compromised quality of life. Ipsilateral loss of taste in the anterior two-third of the tongue, impairment of hearing, reduced lacrimation, and diminished salivary flow of submandibular/sublingual gland are also manifested due to the compromised sensory and parasympathetic innervation of the affected facial nerve.

Diagnosis

- Clinical and imaging evaluation

Extraoral inspection and palpation of the lymph nodes, temporomandibular joints, masticatory muscles, and detailed intraoral screening to map the affected area. Head and neck imaging may be requested to rule out any local or central space occupying lesion or pathology (i.e., sclerotic plaques, strokes, and demyelinating disease).

- Quantitative sensory testing and sialometry
- Blood count and serologic tests

Treatment

Complete recovery has been documented in the majority of those affected, leaving approximately 13% with slight paresis and only 5% with long-term significant facial paralysis. However, immediate initiation of therapeutic interventions is crucial to counteract neuropathic destruction and decrease the probability of long-term morbidities. Oral corticosteroid, such as prednisone at 1–2 mg/kg once a day, and antivirals, like acyclovir 400 mg five times a day for 10 days (in cases suspected to be related herpes simplex or zoster infection), is the recommended treatment regimen. This regimen is most efficacious when initiated within 48 h of the onset of symptoms, if no contraindications existed. If pain accompanied the signs of FP, due to herpes zoster infections or otitis media, analgesics such as nonsteroidal anti-inflammatory medications are recommended.

In cases where recovery could not be achieved with short-term pharmacotherapeutics, other modalities including acupuncture, physiotherapy, electrical muscle stimulation, and facial muscles home exercise have demonstrated partial effectiveness.

Table 24.1 Photobiomodulation parameters suggested for treating Facial Palsy

Wavelength (nm)		NIR: 795–830
Power (mW)		100
Radiant energy (J)		4–10/point
Fluence (J/cm^2)		4
Photonic fluence	($p.J/cm^2$)	≈ 6–6.4
	(Einstein)	≈ 1.3–1.4
Exposure time (s/point)		4–10
Spot location		8 points over the course of the facial nerve
Treatment days		3 days/week for 6 weeks[a]

[a]PBM should be considered as an adjunctive tool to other treatment modalities, such as physiotherapy and facial muscles home exercise

In this context, photobiomodulation (PBM) has been suggested to treat FP given its anti-inflammatory and tissue regeneration effect on peripheral nerves, leading to axonal growth, and myelination. A recent systematic review of randomized clinical trials has demonstrated comparable efficacy of PBM to conventional therapy in patients with trigeminal neuralgia (please see respective chapter). Infrared low-level lasers seem to exert favorable effect due to their depth of penetration that coincides with the nerve's location (Table 24.1). Therefore, PBM, with other supportive modalities such as physiotherapy, seems to be a promising approach to treat FP.

Treatment

- *Systemic Pharmacological Treatment*
  - Corticosteroid drugs (prednisone)
  - Antiviral agents (acyclovir)
  - Analgesics
- *Miscellaneous*
  - Acupuncture
  - Physiotherapy
  - Electrical muscle stimulation
- *Photobiomodulation*

Further Reading

Aditya V. LMN facial palsy in pregnancy: an opportunity to predict preeclampsia-report and review. Case Rep Obstet Gynecol. 2014;2014:626871.

Bosco D, Plastino M, Bosco F, Consoli A, Labate A, Pirritano D, Consoli D, Fava A. Bell's Palsy: a manifestation of prediabetes? Acta Neurol Scand. 2011 Jan;123(1):68–72.

Eviston TJ, Croxson GR, Kennedy PG, Hadlock T, Krishnan AV. Bell's Palsy: aetiology, clinical features and multidisciplinary care. J Neurol Neurosurg Psychiatry. 2015 Dec;86(12):1356–61.

Ibarra AMC, Biasotto-Gonzalez DA, Kohatsu EYI, de Oliveira SSI, Bussadori SK, Tanganeli JPC. Photobiomodulation on trigeminal neuralgia: systematic review. Lasers Med Sci. 2021 Jun;36(4):715–22.

Javaherian M, Attarbashi Moghaddam B, Bashardoust Tajali S, Dabbaghipour N. Efficacy of low-level laser therapy on management of Bell's palsy: a systematic review. Lasers Med Sci. 2020;35:1245–52.

Kandakurti PK, Shanmugam S, Basha SA, Amaravadi SK, Suganthirababu P, Gopal K, George GS. The effectiveness of low-level laser therapy combined with facial expression exercises in patients with moderate-to-severe Bell's Palsy: a study protocol for a randomized controlled trial. Int J Surg Protoc. 2020;24:39–44.

Kennelly KD. Clinical neurophysiology of cranial nerve disorders. Handb Clin Neurol. 2019;161:327–42.

Peng KP, Chen YT, Fuh JL, Tang CH, Wang SJ. Increased risk of Bell palsy in patients with migraine: a nationwide cohort study. Neurology. 2015 Jan 13;84(2):116–24.

Singh A, Deshmukh P. Bell's Palsy: a review. Cureus. 2022 Oct 11;14(10):e30186.

Chapter 25
Temporomandibular Dysfunction

Thaís Cristina Esteves-Pereira, Mariana de Pauli Paglioni, Francisco Javier Tejeda Nava, and Mario Nava-Villalba

Disease Definition

Temporomandibular dysfunction (TMD) is a disorder of the masticatory muscles and/or temporomandibular joints, and it is also the most common cause of pain at the stomatognathic system that is not dental-related. It presents a multifactorial etiology, and its main symptoms include muscular or joint pain, trismus, and alteration of mandibular movements, vertigo, among others. They occur in all age groups, mainly in adults, with a higher incidence in women than men (range of 3:1), mostly at 30 years old. Probably, a cause related to hormones, such as estrogen, may justify such predisposition. Women also have the double of chances to manifest pain when diagnosed with TMD. TMD is considered an important public health problem, because it generally affects negatively patient's daily activities, and its management and treatment may be challenging.

T. C. Esteves-Pereira (✉) · M. de Pauli Paglioni
Oral Diagnosis Department, Piracicaba Dental School, University of Campinas, Piracicaba, SP, Brazil

F. J. T. Nava
Faculty of Stomatology, Autonomous University of San Luis Potosí, San Luis Potosí, Mexico
e-mail: francisco.tejeda@uaslp.mx

M. Nava-Villalba
Pathology Research and Diagnostic Center, Microbiology and Pathology Department, Health Sciences University Center, University of Guadalajara, Guadalajara, JAL, Mexico
e-mail: mario.nava@academicos.udg.mx

A. R. Santos-Silva et al. (eds.), *Photobiomodulation Therapy in Oral Medicine*,
https://doi.org/10.1007/978-3-031-85048-6_25

Diagnosis

- Clinical evaluation. Find below some clinical signs normally associated with TMD:
  1. Dental wear with or without loss of vertical dimension occlusion
  2. Deviation of the chin during opening and closing mandibular movements
  3. Joint displacement during mandibular movements
  4. The others discussed above in "Disease definition"

Treatment

TMD treatment often requires multidisciplinary and multimodalities approaches. Normally, the initial management of TMD is nonsurgical and aims to reduce the level of symptoms. Myorelaxant splints, physiotherapy, pharmaceutical therapies, photobiomodulation (PBM), and others compose the portfolio of treatment for TMD.

PBM stimulates the metabolism of substances involved in analgesia, modulates the inflammation, and involves easy-handling devices, and no contraindication is reported. Mandibular movements may be restored when pain is reduced. Among PBM therapies, LED light presents as a further option in the treatment of TMD. LEDs are semiconductor diodes (p–n junction), which when energized emit light, with advantage of the cost of the device, the possibility of using clusters to irradiate larger areas at a single time, the association of different wavelengths, and absence of side effects. Studies have suggested that LED therapy provides relief of pain, increase in range of motion, and improvement of muscular activity in patients with TMD.

A few clinical trials are available in the current literature for guidance to clinicians regarding PBM parameters. However, there is a significant range between them. Therefore, Table 25.1 and Fig. 25.1 recommendations are based on the most homogenous studies that allowed a statistical analysis, which allows readership to be based on clinical improvements with reduced bias information. Moreover, information should be carefully interpreted by professionals until more clinical trials are performed.

Table 25.1 Photobiomodulation parameters suggested for treating temporomandibular dysfunction

Wavelength (nm)		NIR: 780–910
Power (mW)		100
Radiant energy (J)		4/point
Fluence (J/cm^2)		4
Photonic fluence	(p.J/cm^2)	≈ 5.6–6.4
	(Einstein)	≈ 1.2–1.4
Exposure time (s/point)		40
Spot location		5 points in the regions of the TM joints, 3 points in the regions of the masseter muscles, and 3 points in the anterior portion of the temporal muscles
Treatment days		2–3 sessions/week for 4 weeks[a]

[a]Other treatment approaches should be considered if symptoms are not improved

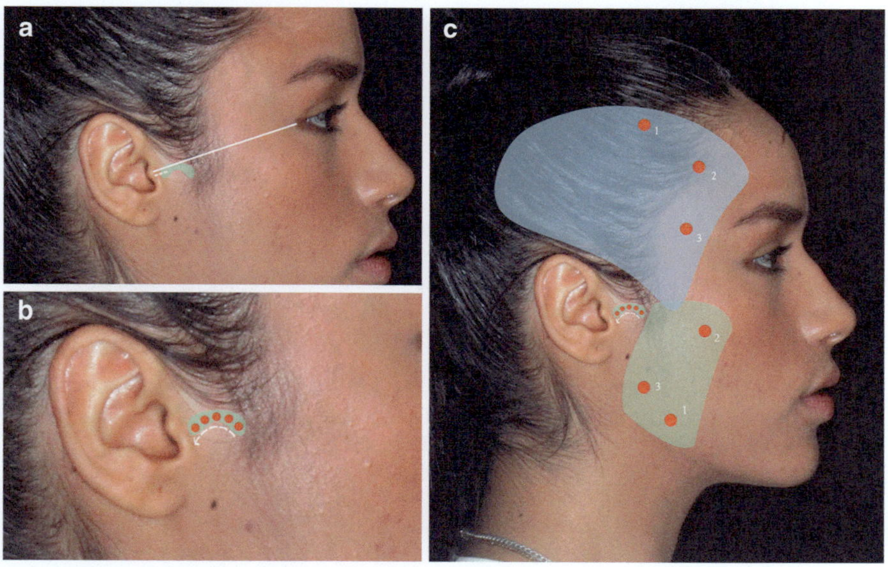

Fig. 25.1 Spot location for the application of the NIR laser protocol described in Table 25.1. (**a**) Location of the TM joint. (**b**) Five application points on each temporomandibular joint. (**c**) Three application points in the anterior temporal muscle region and three application points in the masseter muscle region

Treatment

- *Systemic Pharmacological Treatment*
  - Analgesics
  - Nonsteroidal anti-inflammatory drugs
  - Muscle relaxants
  - Benzodiazepines
  - Antidepressants
- *Surgical treatment*
  - Surgical treatment should be defined by the bucomaxillofacial surgeon
- *Miscellaneous*
  - Occlusal devices
  - Acupuncture
  - Orofacial myofunctional therapy
  - Electrostimulation
- *Photobiomodulation*

Further Reading

Ahmad SA, Hasan S, Saeed S, Khan A, Khan M. Low-level laser therapy in temporomandibular joint disorders: a systematic review. J Med Life. 2021;14:148–64.

Chen J, Huang Z, Ge M, Gao M. Efficacy of low-level laser therapy in the treatment of TMDs: a meta-analysis of 14 randomised controlled trials. J Oral Rehabil. 2015;42:291–9.

Gauer RL, Semidey MJ. Diagnosis and treatment of temporomandibular disorders. Am Fam Physician. 2015;91:378–86.

Máximo CFGP, Coêlho JF, Benevides SD, Alves GÂDS. Effects of low-level laser photobiomodulation on the masticatory function and mandibular movements in adults with temporomandibular disorder: a systematic review with meta-analysis. Codas. 2022;34:e20210138.

Romero-Reyes M, Klasser G, Akerman S. An update on temporomandibular disorders (TMDs) and headache. Curr Neurol Neurosci Rep. 2023 Oct;23(10):561–70.

Shobha R, Narayanan VS, Jagadish Pai BS, Jaishankar HP, Jijin MJ. Low-level laser therapy: a novel therapeutic approach to temporomandibular disorder – a randomized, double-blinded, placebo-controlled trial. Indian J Dent Res. 2017;28:380–7.

Sousa DFM, Gonçalves MLL, Politti F, Lovisetto RDP, Fernandes KPS, Bussadori SK, Mesquita-Ferrari RA. Photobiomodulation with simultaneous use of red and infrared light emitting diodes in the treatment of temporomandibular disorder: study protocol for a randomized, controlled and double-blind clinical trial. Medicine (Baltimore). 2019;98:e14391.

Index

A
Adjunctive therapy, 3
Adverse effects, 27
Antiangiogenic medications, 58
Antimicrobial photodynamic therapy (aPDT), 65, 77, 78, 81, 91
  diagnostic criteria, 79
  different days, 78
  treatment, 80–82

B
Bone-modifying agents (BMA), 55
Burning mouth syndrome (BMS), 111
  diagnosis, 111–113
  glossodynia, 111
  pathogenesis, 112
  photobiomodulation therapy, 114
  treatment, 113, 114

C
Chemotherapy, 41
Cross-infection, 25, 26
Cytochrome c oxidase (Cox), 6, 7

D
Desquamative gingivitis, 104
Disposable barriers, 25, 26
Dosimetry, 11, 13
Dysgeusia, 41, 42
  diagnosis, 42
  treatment, 43

F
Facial palsy (FP), 125
  diagnosis, 126
  neuromotor disorder, 125
  photobiomodulation, 127
  treatment, 126, 127

G
Geographic tongue (GT)
  clinical presentation, 107
  diagnosis, 108
  etiology, 107
  migratory glossitis, 107
  treatment, 108, 109
Graft versus host disease (GvHD), 73
  diagnosis, 74
  hyposalivation, 74
  salivary flow, 75
  treatment, 74, 75

H
Hematopoietic stem cell transplantation (HSCT), 36
Herpes simplex virus (HSV), 125
Hyposalivation, 69, 73, 74
  diagnosis, 69–70
  treatment, 70, 71

I
International Association for the Study of Pain (IASP), 117

A. R. Santos-Silva et al. (eds.), *Photobiomodulation Therapy in Oral Medicine*,
https://doi.org/10.1007/978-3-031-85048-6

International Headache Society (IHS), 111
Intravenous bisphosphonates, 56, 57

L

Light-emitting diodes (LEDs), 17, 18
Lymphedema, 28

M

Medication-related osteonecrosis of the jaw (MRONJ), 55, 81
 diagnosis, 59
 effective management, 59
 incidence, 56
 oral bisphosphonates, 56
 pathogenesis, 55
 treatment, 59, 60
Mucous membrane pemphigoid (MMP), 103
 desquamative gingivitis, 104
 diagnosis, 104
 photobiomodulat, 105
 treatment, 104, 105

N

Neuropathic pain (NP)
 classification, 118
 diagnosis, 118
 orofacial region, 117
 photobiomodulation parameters, 119
 treatment, 118, 119

O

Oral lichen planus (OLP), 95
 chronic mucocutaneous disorder, 95
 diagnosis, 96
 relief of symptoms, 96
 skin manifestations, 96
 treatment, 96, 97
Oral mucositis (OM), 28, 33, 34, 36
 diagnosis, 36
 gastrointestinal tract, 33
 treatment, 37, 38
Oral squamous cell carcinoma (OSCC), 38
Osteoradionecrosis, 63, 64, 81
 diagnosis, 64
 photobiomodulation, 66
 treatment, 65–68

P

Pemphigus vulgaris (PV), 99
 diagnosis, 100
 direct immunofluorescence, 100
 indirect immunofluorescence, 100
 photobiomodulation, 101
 treatment, 100, 101
Pentoxifylline-tocopherol-clodronate combination (PENTOCLO), 52, 65
Peripheral neuropathy, 28
Photobiomodulation (PBM), 3, 5, 6, 18–22, 26, 28, 38, 43, 66, 67, 70, 82, 87, 92, 97, 105, 108, 113, 119, 123
 clinical efficacy, 5
 dosimetry, 11
 mechanisms, 9
 parameters, 12–13
 primary effect, 6, 7
 protocol, 11
 radiosensitivity, 17
 secondary effect, 7, 8
 tertiary effect, 8, 9
 wavelength, 13
Photosensitizing agent (PA), 77

R

Radiation dermatitis (RD), 49
 diagnosis, 50
 photobiomodulation, 52
 treatment, 50–52
Radiodermatitis, 28
Radiotherapy, 41, 70
Ramsay Hunt syndrome, 125
RANK ligand inhibitor (denosumab), 58
Reactive oxygen species (ROS), 7
Recurrent aphthous stomatitis (RAS), 85, 86
 diagnosis, 86
 endocrine imbalance, 86
 gastrointestinal condition, 86
 photobiomodulation, 87
 treatment, 86, 87
Recurrent herpes labialis (RHL), 89, 90
 diagnosis, 90
 HSV-1, 89
 photobiomodulation, 92
 treatment, 91, 92

T

Targeted therapy, 41
Taste alteration, 41

Temporomandibular dysfunction (TMD), 129
  diagnosis, 130
  muscular activity, 130
  photobiomodulation, 131
  treatment, 130, 132
Tic douloureux, 121
Tissue surface irradiance (TSI), 14
Trigeminal neuralgia (TN), 118, 121
  diagnosis, 122
  head and neck region, 121
  photobiomodulation, 123
  tic douloureux, 121
  treatment, 122, 123
  vascular compression, 122
Trismus, 45
  diagnosis, 46
  mouth opening, 45
  photobiomodulation, 46
  treatment, 46, 47

V
Visual analogue scale (VAS), 46

W
Wound healing, 87

X
Xerostomia, 112

MIX
Papier aus verantwortungsvollen Quellen
Paper from responsible sources
FSC® C105338

If you have any concerns about our products,
you can contact us on
ProductSafety@springernature.com

In case Publisher is established outside the EU,
the EU authorized representative is:
Springer Nature Customer Service Center GmbH
Europaplatz 3, 69115 Heidelberg, Germany

Printed by Libri Plureos GmbH
in Hamburg, Germany